MUSIC

ARTS FOR HEALTH

Series Editor: Paul Crawford, Professor of Health Humanities, University of Nottingham, UK

The *Arts for Health* series offers a ground-breaking set of books that guide the general public, carers and healthcare providers on how different arts can help people to stay healthy or improve their health and wellbeing.

Bringing together new information and resources underpinning the health humanities (that link health and social care disciplines with the arts and humanities), the books demonstrate the ways in which the arts offer people worldwide a kind of shadow health service – a non-clinical way to maintain or improve our health and wellbeing. The books are aimed at general readers along with interested arts practitioners seeking to explore the health benefits of their work, health and social care providers and clinicians wishing to learn about the application of the arts for health, educators in arts, health and social care and organizations, carers and individuals engaged in public health or generating healthier environments. These easy-to-read, engaging short books help readers to understand the evidence about the value of arts for health and offer guidelines, case studies and resources to make use of these non-clinical routes to a better life.

Other titles in the series:

Film	Steven Schlozman
Theatre	Sydney Cheek-O'Donnell
Singing	Yoon Irons and Grenville Hancox
Reading	Philip Davis
Drawing	Curie Scott
Photography	Susan Hogan
Storytelling	Michael Wilson

Forthcoming titles:

Gaming and Game Design	Sandra Danilovic
History	Anna Greenwood
Painting	Javier Saaavedra, Samuel Arias, and Ana Rodríguez
Magic	Richard Wiseman

Music and the arts reach around all corners of the world and into all corners of our life and Dr Eugene Beresin details many aspects of their purpose and importance in his book *Arts For Health: Music*. I think this is important information to share and it reinforces what all of us musicians and artists already know…that the arts (regardless of their type), when done with the right intention, are healing arts.

– Jeff Coffin, 3x Grammy winning saxophonist, composer, educator, author. Dave Matthews Band, Bela Fleck & the Flecktones, Ear Up Records founder, The Mu'tet.

Music is certainly a pleasurable and universal part of the human experience, but is it really possible that harms could be assuaged through harmonies, symptoms soothed by symphonies, remedies found in rhythm? As an expert Harvard physician, healer, and musician, Dr Gene Beresin makes a forceful and persuasive case that the answer is a resounding, "yes" – scientifically elucidating and affirming music's psycho-biological therapeutic effects and uncovering its power to heal. Informative, instructive, inspirational, students, clinicians, patients, and family members, will find solace and joy here.

– John F. Kelly, PhD, ABPP Elizabeth R. Spallin Professor of Psychiatry in Addiction Medicine, Harvard Medical School, Director of the Recovery Research Institute, Massachusetts General Hospital, Boston, MA, USA. Award-winning songwriter, singer, musician, and producer.

If you are in the group of people that think music is ancillary to your life – or extracurricular or non-essential – but have been waiting for someone to prove you wrong, look no further! Dr Eugene Beresin has comprehensively, and in simple language, dispelled any hypothesis of the kind in his book, *Arts For Health: Music*. From heartfelt personal testimonies to factual medical data, this book beautifully explains the effect music universally has on humanity and why it's important for individual well-being. It is a must have for all music teachers, students and professionals, as it gives language to what we innately already know.

– Terri Lyne Carrington – Grammy Award winning, drummer/composer/producer/activist, who is played with Herbie Hancock, Wayne Shorter, Stan Getz, Al Jarreau and many others.

Music has a visceral, transcendent power that cuts across language, culture and age, and it can help us connect to each other, as well as to our innermost selves. In Arts For Health: Music, Gene Beresin has created a fantastic reminder of and argument for music's power to lead us to healthier, more connected, and more fulfilling lives.

— *Chris Eldridge – Grammy winning acoustic guitarist with Punch Brothers, Julian Lage. Americana Music Association Instrumentalist of the Year. Visiting Assistant Professor of Contemporary Acoustic Music, Oberlin Conservatory.*

MUSIC

EUGENE BERESIN
The Massachusetts General Hospital and
Harvard Medical School, USA

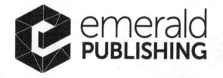

United Kingdom – North America – Japan – India
Malaysia – China

Emerald Publishing Limited
Howard House, Wagon Lane, Bingley BD16 1WA, UK

First edition 2022

British Library Cataloguing in Publication Data
A catalogue record for this book is available from the British
Library

ISBN: 978-1-83867-316-1 (Print)
ISBN: 978-1-83867-313-0 (Online)
ISBN: 978-1-83867-315-4 (Epub)

ISOQAR certified
Management System,
awarded to Emerald
for adherence to
Environmental
standard
ISO 14001:2004.

ISOQAR
REGISTERED
Certificate Number 1985
ISO 14001

INVESTOR IN PEOPLE

This book is dedicated to my mother, Marcella Grace Beresin, who inspired my love of music and playing by ear. I was no match for her performance of Chopin's Fantaisie Impromptu.

CONTENTS

SERIES PREFACE:
CREATIVE PUBLIC HEALTH

The "Arts for Health" series aims to provide key information on how different arts and humanities practices can support, or even transform, health and wellbeing. Each book introduces a particular creative activity or resource and outlines its place and value in society, the evidence for its use in advancing health and wellbeing, and cases of how this works. In addition, each book provides useful links and suggestions to readers for following-up on these quick reads. We can think of this series as a kind of shadow health service – encouraging the use of the arts and humanities alongside all the other resources on offer to keep us fit and well.

Creative practices in the arts and humanities offer a fantastic, non-medical, but medically relevant way to improve the health and wellbeing of individuals, families and communities. Intuitively, we know just how important creative activities are in maintaining or recovering our best possible lives. For example, imagine that we woke up tomorrow to find that all music, books or films had to be destroyed, learn that singing, dancing or theatre had been outlawed or that galleries, museums and theatres had to close permanently; or, indeed, that every street had posters warning citizens of severe punishment for taking photographs, drawing or writing. How would we feel? What would happen to our bodies and minds? How would we survive? Unfortunately, we have seen this kind of removal of creative activities from human society before and today many people remain terribly restricted in artistic expression and consumption.

I hope that this series adds a practical resource to the public. I hope people buy these little books as gifts for family and friends, or for hard-pressed healthcare professionals, to encourage them to revisit or to consider a creative path to living well. I hope that creative public health makes for a brighter future.

Professor Paul Crawford

ACKNOWLEDGMENTS

I am deeply grateful to so many people who gracefully put up with my obsessive and repetitive questions and commentary about the content of this book – mostly my wife Michaela and my children, Jade, Caitlin, Glennon and Zack, along with their partners. I could not have produced this manuscript without the support and encouragement from the staff of the Clay Center for Young Healthy Minds at MGH both for the production of this book and for my intense focus on writing sound-tracks. I am indebted to my dear friends in our Band, Pink Freud and the Transitional Objects – David, Tony, Brad, Boz, Bill, Chris, and Kari, who continually inspire my playing and writing music. You are the backbone of a communal process that keeps my musical sensibilities alive and growing. Thank you. I am indebted to Paul Crawford for allowing me the time to write, extension after extension, as I had to deal with the pandemic through my work at the Clay Center and with my MGH medical students, residents, and patients. And I would be lost without my teachers Ben Cook and Earl Pughe, who gently and relentlessly push me to the limit on piano and guitar. Thank you all.

1

WHY MUSIC? THE UNIVERSALITY OF MUSIC

"I don't sing because I'm happy. I'm happy because I sing."

William James

We are all immersed in music. From the time we get up in the morning, uncomfortably listening to the radio alarm we have set to music, to a venture to the mall, enduring the background music to a pop up on our computers, or watching TV – commercials, soundtracks for movies and series, to firing up our personal playlists. Music is ubiquitous. This is not to say we always pay attention to it, but it is inescapable.

Dick Clark, the creator and host of American Bandstand famously said, "music is the soundtrack of your life." And in many ways, it is.

But beyond our immersion, by choice or by chance, music is universal as we will argue below, and serves a multiplicity of functions in our lives.

THE PLACE OF MUSIC IN HUMAN SOCIETY

Let's look at the many places and functions of music in our lives.

1. Reinforcing Social and Community Cohesion and Rituals:
  Music plays a core role in religious and spiritual services, and

this is true for all cultures. It is instrumental in coordination with scriptures, whether sung by a religious leader, to a chorus, to the community singing together. It serves to honor births, deaths, and holidays.

Music is fundamental in transmitting cultural rituals universally, such as drum circles, tribal dances, weddings (and, of course, in some cultures, the rituals of the first dance of a marital couple, to the dance with mother or father). The history of a culture is often depicted in song with or without lyrics. Music is fundamental in connecting people in a community. Concerts are a superb example of our feeling a compelling sense of connection, not just to the band but to each other.

And furthermore, music is inherently social. Music is deeply embedded in our social structure. All the examples above involve a social context. Even when you sing in the shower, you typically have an audience in mind. The context of all musical performances, solo or collective involves social relationships.

2. **Supporting Relationships:** Music is listened to in families, among lovers, with friends, with parents and kids of all ages. Some tunes are unique and special between siblings, parents, grandparents, or romantic partners. Remember your favorite dance tune – one that you and your friends, got up and danced together? It was a joyous group experience. Most of us hearken back to a tune that is special for unique (often teenage) relationships. Music is the glue that binds us, reminds us of times that were upsetting or uplifting, but in the context of relationships, the most powerful medium that strengthens our interpersonal connections.

3. **Solidifying Identity:** In a similar fashion, music, often specific genres, songs, lyrics have special meaning to adolescents and young adults – earmarking and becoming emblematic of their identity. During those seminal years of high school and young adulthood, there is a fundamentally important place songs hold in personal and collective identity formation.

4. **Evoking Feelings and Attendant Memories:** Music is probably among the most powerful stimuli that stirs emotions. It makes

us feel happy, sad, scared, makes us want to get up and dance or clap our hands. This is perhaps the greatest power of music. And many tunes evoke memories associated with the music – memories of music at your special birthday party, at the prom or sadly, at a funeral. We all can recall a tune symbolic of an important event. Remember your first romantic partner, and "our song"? Even though they broke up with you, and you were devastated, when you hear that special song, you smile as it brings you back to driving in the car with them. Many of our old memories are associated with music. This is one way that folks with dementia sharpen their autobiographical memory when they hear songs of the childhood. Long-term memory certainly remains beyond loss of short term, and music may well be the trigger of earlier life experience.

5. **Triggering Movement:** Who can listen to gospel music, or attend a rock concert without tapping your feet, clapping your hands, or wanting to get up and dance. There is an intrinsic component of music as we will see in its neurobiology, that is linked to rhythm, dance, and drumming. Music is inherently physical, and the combination of playing, listening, singing, and dancing has been fundamental to all cultures. Music's rhythmic structure and tempo are intrinsically powerful. We will see how the combination of music and dance has profound therapeutic potential (as well as intense synergy) for our enjoyment.

6. **Accentuating the Value of Hymns and Anthems:** A particular place of music in society is it's symbolizing a specialized group. Common examples include national anthems, university fight songs, most often supporting their athletic teams, and military marches. Many tear up when they hear *America the Beautiful*, the *Star-Spangled Banner* or *Anchors Away*. It stirs up con- nection to something we treasure as a community, but it also brings tears to our eyes, if we hear the national anthem at a baseball game we powerfully recall when our mom or dad took us to the ballgame. Much of this reminds us of seminal events in our lives and amplifies our emotional responses of elation, drama, loss, or other evocative events we never forget.

Another function of the anthem is to amplify the history of nations, communities, spiritual and cultural groups, movements, or organizations by calling up special events and missions through the integration of narrative and poetic pieces. This often evokes elation, nostalgia, or melancholy. For example, the songs of Woody Guthrie remind us about the perils of immigration, the migration West, the losses from the Dust Bowl, and the formation of Unions. His music documented the adversity of his times, and the toll it took on sectors of the population. The chants of slaves on the chain gang helped offset the emotional and physical burdens, distracting them from pain, and at the same time provided a means for their bonding against oppression. In that light, music has served to stir emotions, and associate groups of people with missions – like the folk songs of protest in the 1960s.

7. **Amplifying and Coloring Other Art Forms:** When was the last time you saw a film without a soundtrack? Music adds coloration, mood, character, and amplification of action to film in powerful (or subtle) ways. Music makes Broadway shows come alive, and often we remember the tunes more than the plot. So, too in dance, opera, circuses, and other forms of performance art. They rely on music as a fundamental part of the art form. Musical themes often represent characters, like Grandpa in Peter and the Wolf, or the Wicked Witch of the West (you know she is coming when you hear the music!)

8. **Fostering Personal Expression and Communication with Others:** Individual expression through music and dance may be accomplished collectively or individually. When we sing together, play music together, or dance together something special happens. The whole is greater than the sum of its parts. We simultaneously can connect with ourselves (no one dances the same as anyone else!) and bond with others. Personal expression, on the other hand, is embodied in a solo improvisation on an instrument, or a solo verse in a song. And it is the epitome of communicating with others. For example, in many tunes, trading 4s or 8s (each person taking a solo for 4 or 8 measures) is

common in jazz. And call and answer is a cornerstone of many tunes, especially seen in songs supporting a collective mission, from chain gangs, to protest songs to hymns in church. Turn taking allows all of us to join in the song. In *The Weight*, by The Band, for example, each verse is sung by a band member, and the chorus is performed collectively in harmony. Writing music for yourself or others, with or without lyrics, is a clear statement of who you are and how you are feeling.

9. **Managing Emotions:** Music has been clearly demonstrated to significantly influence our emotional states. This ranges from fostering soothing attachments between parents and infants through lullabies, to passive listening of music preparing for medical procedures, to simply listening to your playlist with friends or alone, when you need to modify your anger, sadness, or simply feel calmer. The power of music to evoke, quell, or amplify emotions is well documented.

10. **Promoting Distraction:** Sometimes music is used to help us divert our attention. As we will see, in pre- and post-operative states, music is extremely effective in reducing anxiety and pain. In addition, it may help distract us from emotional upset and/or trauma by re-directing our attention, for example, if we didn't do a great job on an exam, or in the workplace; or if we had a fight with a partner. Sometimes, we use music to re-direct our feelings.

11. **Improving Cognition and Coordination:** Music lessons can help kids (and later adults) improve many aspects of their thinking and motor skills. For patients with dementia, the same is true, as we will see below in the Chapter 2. For some kids with Autistic Spectrum Disorder, music may be beneficial in communication, social interactions and diminishing stereotypic behavior, such as hand flapping. And for older folks, it has shown to help cognitive functions, and diminish movement disorders in Parkinson's Disease. For younger kids, music has helped learn numbers, new languages, colors and more. Sesame Street and its clever songs enhance learning.

DEFINING HEALTH AND WELL-BEING

Without being utterly pedantic, I want us to think about how we define "health" and "well-being." The World Health Organization (WHO) defines health as "a state of complete physical, mental and social well-being and not merely the absence of disease or infirmity" (Fancourt & Finn, 2019). Before we can figure out how music can enhance these states of being, they need some clarification.

What is so valuable about this definition is that it acknowledges that health does not rule out the presence of illness (MacDonald et al., 2012). After all, we all have some illness, and one can be "healthy" despite having diabetes, cardiovascular illness, depression, or another physical infirmity. Furthermore, it indicates that health is not simply dependent on the professional treatment of clinicians, but may be fostered, despite illness, by social, emotional, cultural, or creative arts. Thus, taking health out of the hands of professional caregivers broadens the concept tremendously (MacDonald, 2013).

However, neither here nor in much of the medical or health-related literature is well-being defined. I think this requires attention, particularly if we intend to see how music can enhance so-called well-being.

PERMA AND PERMA +4

Seligman defines the framework of well-being as involving: Positive Emotions, Engagement, Relationships, Meaning, and Accomplishments (**PERMA**). This has become the cornerstone of the school of positive psychology. Briefly, **Positive emotions** can come to the fore from the past, present and hope for the future. **Engagement** is one's application of skills to challenging tasks. **Relationships** are our connection with others, and bring us support, comfort, enjoyment, and the ability if needed to resolve conflict. They also provide us with a sense of belonging, so we do not feel alone. **Meaning** is how we value our purpose and role in family, spiritual groups, community, work, and take pride in our role and place within these structures. And finally, **Accomplishments** are how we view our sense of mastery, achievement in any domain (Seligman, 2002).

Well-being is highly individualized. This is super important! We each work and take on these building blocks to a greater or lesser degree. Well-being is viewed as a dynamic and ongoing mission that offers us greater and greater satisfaction. We all use different tools to attain higher levels of each building block – and music is one of many. Research has shown that the more we attain higher degrees of well-being within these domains, we improve our overall health, daily functioning, emotional state, sense of identity, personal pride, and competence among other attributes.

Seligman was criticized that **PERMA** did not include some very important elements that are vital for well-being, and hence the development of **PERMA +4** (Seligman, 2018). This would include Physical Health, Mindset, Work Environment, and Economic Security. **Physical Health** includes the highest levels of biological assets, such as optimal sleep, diet, nutrition, as well as high levels of functioning despite physical limitations, often due to illness. **Mindset** is defined as a "growth" mindset – the belief that one's abilities and talents can develop over time, and that we can learn from our failures. **Work Environment** involves the physical, social, and cultural features of our workplace and how we cope with them. All of us are influenced by the context within which we work. Hopefully, awareness of deficits in the workplace will motive us to foster change. Finally, **Economic Security** was added as it is well-established that financial matters are a strong predictor of well-being. To the extent we can have control over our financial situation, make reasonable decisions that are responsible for ourselves and our families, and strive to improve our economic status, our well-being will improve (Donaldson & Ellardus van Zyl, 2022).

What I like about this multidimensional model is that it is fluid, and considers the individual's role, emotional and mental state, social role, and the influence of community in its broadest sense in achieving well-being (Iasiello et al., 2017). Thus, one might literally be dying, in palliative care, and with sufficient elements of PERRL +4, be in a state of positive well-being. By the same token, a person of great economic means, with all the social and material benefits, at least superficially, might have far lower well-being. Like everything else, it's all relative.

I am taking the time to delineate these elements of well-being because they are all interconnected, but if music can enhance any one or more of them, we can improve health. I think the most powerful testimony to the individuality of well-being and the ways music enhances our physical and mental conditions, is reading the personal and intimate vignettes of a several individuals in Chapter 3, considering what we can do to implement the benefits of music. Please keep PERMA+4 in mind.

THE ROLE OF HAPPINESS IN WELL-BEING

Isn't it odd that nothing above connected well-being to happiness? After all, if you are in a pretty good state of well-being, you should be happy, right? And for most of us, music, even sad music, makes us happy. So, shouldn't it contribute to well-being?

The Dali Lama, in a keynote at the 7th Global Spa & Wellness Summit (April 2022), noted that

> *happiness is the key to overall wellness. There are a few things that are necessary to achieve a happy life apart from physical wellbeing and these include* a happy mind, compassion, trust, friendship, and affection. *(Dali Lama, 2013)*

While we could consider compassion, trust, friendship, and affection as a part of healthy relationships, the key addition to our concept of well-being is having a happy mind. Happiness is an independent variable, given the PERMA +4 components above. For example, you can suffer from a chronic physical illness, have difficulty engaging in challenges, failed accomplishments, but offset by positive relationships, social supports, and perhaps with the use of music as one of the creative arts in our toolbox, have a happy mind. If your mindset, the compassion and affection from others, among other variables line up, you can feel happy. It is not easy, but it is attainable. We need happiness as an overall goal for well-being.

Remember that health and well-being are not static or linear. We all have our ups and downs. When bad things happen, we dip in our sense of well-being. Thus, efforts at being resilient, and having means to bounce back is of vital importance. As I hope to show, music, among other creative arts, is one way to reclaim our sense of well-being.

THE NEUROBIOLOGY OF MUSIC

According to Levitin (2006) among others our brains are wired at birth to respond to music. As he points out there is no one center that provides all the processing functions of music but rather, a complex network of regions of the brain, serving different purposes, and a system of neurotransmitters (the chemicals that transmit messages from one neuron to another), that are particularly prominent in the response to music (Chanda & Levitin, 2013). As he points out, when we listen to music, a cascade of brain regions are activated in a particular order. First, the auditory cortex processes the sound after music is heard by the ear, followed by the regions in the frontal part of the brain that organize musical structure and experiences. We also get input from the mesolimbic system (the part of the brain involved in arousal and pleasure), the transmission of key "reward" chemicals, production of opioids and dopamine, finally activating the nucleus accumbens (the center of the brain's reward system) (Blood & Zatorre, 2001). This is all supported by the cerebellum (the very back part of the brain) that regulates emotion by its focus on rhythm, and its connection to the frontal lobe and limbic system (that also contributes to emotional states, and memory, linking conscious and unconscious parts of our brain). Levitin also has postulated that music improves well-being through neurochemical systems for reward, motivation, stress, and arousal.

Another way of looking at it is this: Our brain pathways associated with musical responses are: (1) Euphoria/pleasant emotion pathways; (2) Reward pathways; (3) Arousal pathways; and (4) Evaluation of reward/punishment pathways (Bostic et al., 2019). For our purposes, it is not as important to know all the neurological structures involved, but rather that our brains are wired to appreciate (or dislike) music. We are born with these capabilities, just as Chomsky noted long ago that our brains are pre-wired to use and understand speech. Thus, music and speech are primed at birth for input, then, depending on the input, will respond, make sense of it, and use for personal and social purposes. This, in large part contributes to the universality of music – our intrinsic wiring that allows for our evaluation of music as positive, negative, arousing, or calming.

THE UNIVERSALITY OF MUSIC

While our brains may be wired to process and appreciate music, many have noted that this does not account for the "universality" of music. Although all cultures have created music, it is quite different across the globe and has changed drastically over time. This has led some scholars to note that though our brains are wired in similar fashions, how is the song (music with lyrics), universal? After all, we are all wired to play various sports, and yet they are vastly different in different cultures. So, if truly universal, what is the common denominator?

In a recent article in the journal, *Science*, the authors examined written accounts of music from over 100 years, including 315 societies. They found that the form of the music in all cultures is universally common in terms of its emotional and behavioral effects. Furthermore, they determined that there is much greater variability within each culture than across cultures. What is common across cultures? Each song event is characterized by different degrees of formality, arousal (level of excitement) and religiosity. And these three areas are regularly defined for purposes of dance, healing, love, and lullaby. The way the accent, tempo, quality of pitch collection, tone, rhythm, and other musical structures such as intervals, variations, etc. are used, defines the purpose and function of the song (Mehr et al., 2019).

Here is how it works: generally, dance songs are high in formality, high in arousal and low religiosity. Healing songs have high formality, high arousal, and high religiosity. Love songs cluster in low formality, low arousal, and low formality and finally, lullabies have low formality, low arousal, and low religiosity. They determined the nature of formality, arousal and religiosity based on many descriptions of tone, pitch, tempo, rhythm, and other musical elements from all these societies. As noted, while these structural features are common between different cultures, their melodies for example, may vary greatly. And within a culture, the different types of say dance tunes may vary greatly between cultures, the basic structures are the same.

Why is this important? It means that there may be common ways the brain is wired in people all over the globe such that they process and use music in the same ways. And by using song, it combines the common wiring hypothesis of Chomsky and Levitin. It adds to the picture that all cultures around the world for all time, have used song for similar purposes – in this case dance, healing, love, and infant care. It makes sense.

This finding is important because it means that our use of music for healing, soothing and dance, for example, may be universal and applicable to individuals regardless of their ethnic or cultural origin.

Additional arguments note that the pentatonic scale consisting of five notes, developed by ancient civilizations, occurs in almost every culture on earth with some variation (https://www.percussionplay.com/five five-notes-to-rule-them-all/). Another theory of universality is that pitch intervals (the space between two notes) convey emotion. And that the intervals used in speech and music, when similar convey the same emotion. The most common example of this is the descending minor third interval (three notes apart) is heard in both speech and music as "sad" across cultural groups (Curtis & Bharucha, 2010), and the emotion of anger is heard by the dissonant ascending second (two notes apart). These findings have been used to demonstrate the universality of music, and how common use of speech, tonality, and other elements of vocalization promote the attachment of infants and mothers in all cultures (Leciere et al., 2014). It should be noted that not all music theorists and ethnomusicologists agree with any of these postulated theories of the universality of music.

2

HOW MUSIC IMPROVES
WELL-BEING

In this chapter, we will explore what music helps in mental health and physical health. But before we consider this, it is important to appreciate that there are several ways music is experienced by patients, how it affects them, and what it can do for all of us in everyday life. Let's start with some core definitions.

Music Therapy: According to the American Music Therapy Association, Music Therapy is "the clinical & evidence-based use of music interventions to accomplish individualized goals within a therapeutic relationship by a credentialed professional who has completed an approved music therapy program" (American Music Therapy Association https://www.musictherapy.org/about/musictherapy/). Music therapy interventions can address a variety of healthcare & educational goals:

- Promote Wellness

- Manage Stress

- Alleviate Pain

- Express Feelings

- Enhance Memory

- Improve Communication

- Promote Physical Rehabilitation

Music Medicine: The use of pre-recorded music to improve clinical status before, during or after medical treatment.

Community Music: The process of bringing people together to help them use music to cope with a wide range of physical disabilities, mental disorders, combat inactivity, and provide a means to form social bonds that reduce isolation and loneliness.

Individual Use of Music: While not a formally designated model, vast number of individuals use music on their own to improve their emotional state, physical abilities, and cognition. And most of us simply listen to music because it is intrinsically enjoyable.

Although the implementation of any particular technique is different, e.g., participatory activity, passive listening, solo or group focus, the goals above in music therapy all appear to apply.

A WORD ABOUT EVIDENCE AND RESEARCH

There have been a number of papers critical of a clear scientific basis validating the efficacy of musical interventions to improve health. Some scholars have noted that conclusions are drawn, despite heterogeneity in research methods, small numbers of subjects and variable means of assessing outcomes of musical interventions. Further, many note the paucity of Randomized Controlled Trials (RTCs) to demonstrate the therapeutic effects of music in healthcare. The RCT is a quantitative method (meaning we are seeking numerical or percent responses, usually based on outcome scales), in which one set of subjects is assigned the intervention, and the other, the control group, does not receive the intervention. Typically, the researchers are "blind" to who is in each group, and simply look at the responses to the intervention. It is argued that this method is the best way to eliminate (or reduce) research bias and is considered the "gold standard" of scientific inquiry in medicine.

The RCT is only one of many research methodologies. For example, there are longitudinal studies looking at an intervention and changes over time; there are pilot studies, looking at an intervention with rating scales that are short term; we also have case reports. And perhaps most importantly, there is the use of Qualitative Research that is a naturalistic method that considers the "why" of a social phenomenon rather than the "what." It considers the complex elements contribute to an intervention, using narrative reports of subjects, observations, and focus groups, that undergo rigorous analysis of responses to open-ended questions about a situation or intervention studied. Many in medicine have taken issue with the validity and reliability of qualitative analysis and in most medical literature, it is rarely used, or seen as a second-class citizen, and is considered as not having the same or even remotely comparable value as the RCT. The RCT, for example, has considered which form of musical intervention, Music Therapy, Music Medicine, or Community Music (not to mention individuals who listen or play music alone) has superior outcomes, often defined as a single attainable behavioral goal. In most cases the conclusion is the same: there are insufficient data, and far too many heterogeneous methods for us to come to any conclusions about the efficacy of music in health.

Let us consider musical interventions. Is the RCT the optimal vehicle for inquiry? Or given the complexity of music – its social, communal, and personal meaning – is the complexity and inherent social context more amenable to qualitative analysis as a means of study? I only raise this because many reviews and "meta-analysis" (taking multiple studies, making comparisons, and drawing conclusions) have limited the research to RCT. I would argue that depending on the phenomenon studied, we need both. For example, when looking at overall well-being of residents using music therapy in a nursing home, I would argue qualitative methods are superior. When we consider the criteria for well-being as defined in Chapter 1, there is a significant subjective component to many of the PERMA +4 indicators, and this may not be discerned by quantitative analysis used in RCT. If we want to know if a music therapy intervention decreases tremor in Parkinson's Disease, regardless of the patient's perception and feelings of well-being, we might consider a RCT. I am concerned about this issue, because many have argued that music in health has a rather weak evidentiary base, and this needs to be taken with a grain of salt, as this conclusion is based on the few RCT studies, and not the wealth of other methodologies, that may tell us more about the social-emotional impact of music on individuals and groups.

But let us consider another way of looking at the use of music as a means of promoting well-being. While methods and outcomes are important and we certainly need more rigorous ways of evaluating which technique works best under which circumstances, (including specific outcomes, as well as perceptions of individuals), particularly if we are setting up a large program in a hospital system of care, perhaps we should consider what is common between these musical interventions and reframe our notion of outcomes and limit our focus regarding well-being.

As we have seen well-being as defined by the World Health Organization (WHO) (Fancourt & Finn, 2019), it does not specify any means of evaluating outcome. In fact, their references are a comprehensive blend of diverse methodologies.

The achievement of any component of well-being is to a large extent based on the personal report of an individual or group. If it achieved, and grounded in subjective experience, that is all we need to have achieved our goal. I want to emphasize that the state of well-being, and each of its components, is unique to each individual, group, or community.

Just as one person may respond to a particular intervention and not another, say one antihistamine versus another for allergies or one non-steroidal anti-inflammatory drug for pain, we can accept the value of the one that works. But some might say that this is placebo response. Certainly, in some cases it is. Placebo is a real effect – likely the influence of the brain controlling a specific symptom or complex of symptoms, and regardless of how it works – it works! I want to make this point here because as we will see in the next chapter, the personal narratives of many individuals, their achievement of well-being through the use of music, is highly specific to the person, and we need to accept their reports as sound. The narratives are not part of a RCT, but they are valid, reliable, albeit as single reports. Consider each one as a case report.

Health Musicking: The concept of health Musicking, introduced by Stige, (Bonde, 2011) is a good way to consider the options we all have for using music to improve well-being. Health musicking can be considered as the use of music experiences to regulate emotion, improve social bonding, and bolster cognitive or physical conditions. It can be accomplished by lay-therapists, community practices, or professionals, trained as music therapists, or by health professionals that use music (Bonde, 2011). Rund sees health musicking, apart from dealing with a specific physical condition, as a cultural phenomenon that has specific benefits: agency (sense of mastery), belonging (social connections), vitality (emotional and esthetic enhancement), and meaning (inherent value of the activity and hope) (Ruud, 1997).

How do we decide, then on the model and method we use for our patients, family members community or ourselves? Stige argues that we need to consider (1) *Arena*. That is the location of musical activities that would be optimal, e.g., home, nursing home, hospital service. (2) *Agenda*. This involves the evaluation of the goals, values, and themes that are chosen. (3) *Agents*. This refers to the actors involved in the music-making – in hospital, home, or a community setting. It requires the individual to consider passive, active or participatory use of music. (4) *Activities*. Does the individual want to sing, to improvise, to be a choral member? Is performing what they are considering, or do they want to listen, and if so, listen to prescribed music or preferred music of their choice? (5) *Artefacts*. Music involves instruments, songs, or lyrics (Stige, 2012). And if, for example, instruments, which ones? How do we foster choices? This is up to the individual, family, health care professional in consultation. There is no one-size fits all. Music interventions and the choice of a wide varieties of possibilities is a personal matter of choice, or if the patient cannot choose, then perhaps a health care proxy who knows what they like.

The intrinsic value of Musicking is that it requires that patients, clinicians, family members, clergy, community and virtually anyone in the life of the patient, including the patient themselves, take an active role in consideration of the modality of music (if any) that is being considered.

MUTUAL RECOVERY AND CREATIVE PRACTICE

The medical model has dominated healthcare practices, namely a clinician making a diagnosis and then delivering evidence-based care to the patient. This unidirectional, commodity-based model (note that we call the subject with an illness a patient, and the healthcare professional a provider) may well be used in music therapy, music medicine, and community music, if a leader is established. An alternative model, in concert with true collaborative and preventative care, is the concept of mutual recovery (Crawford et al., 2013). This model that may seem revolutionary to some, is grounded on what many of us as clinicians have long known, yet most have often not admitted – patients and their care have a significant impact on our well-being. The consequences of our engagement in healthcare involve the "recovery" or emotional effects on both the patient and the caregiver. The outcome of our work for better or worse, has an emotional effect on each of us. Thus, the medical model based on long established norms that we "deliver" care and are trained not to look at our own sense of impact by the clinical situation, (or suppress or deny any impact) is radically transformed by considering that clinical care has a profound mutual effect on the patient as well as the clinician.

Some have argued that this is a slippery slope leading to "boundary" infractions. Or that medical training, teaches us not to let our own feelings and reactions enter the clinical arena, lest it interfere with the provision of care, just as it would in caring for a beloved relative. Yet in psychiatry, we know that if we do not process our own emotional reactions to patients, both positive and negative, care suffers. In technical terms, it is appreciating the transference and countertransference in our work. In recent years, many clinicians have suffered from excessive stress, isolation, and burnout. This has been evident long before the COVID pandemic with increased caseloads and clinical demands but has taken on new levels of intensity in the last two years. I would argue that not considering the impact of patient care on the caregiver, has led us to an often untenable situation in many systems of care. This has been dramatically demonstrated in the COVID pandemic and the devastating negative effects on caregivers.

Hence, I would like us to consider the incorporation of mutual recovery into musicking. There are strikingly few references in the literature to this phenomenon, but the handful of work leads us to a better model, particularly for musicking. A nice summary is provided in the WHO report (Fancourt & Finn, 2019, p. 28). And beyond that, I would argue that considering care as a two-way street results in improved treatment and mutual well-being. After all, do we not all benefit from the music that surrounds us in clinical situations? As we read on about what helps, and who is helped (clinical narratives) I encourage you to think about how we need to re-define the "provision" of care (as if it were some kind of commodity) and reframe it as the mutual experience of care in the context of a true collaboration in the domains of agreeing upon treatment plans, locus of care, and the professionals and family or proxies involved.

A. MENTAL HEALTH

Mental health problems are quite amenable to music interventions. Most of us feel mood improving simply by listening to music, particular familiar music that has positive memories associated, or new music by artists we have long appreciated or even discovered in recent years. I would like to address issues and situations that include and go beyond diagnosis. For example, I will consider how music enhances social bonding across the lifespan from infants to the elderly; diminishes loneliness; enhances identity formation; and improves peri-natal conditions. In addition, music has been demonstrated to diminish symptoms of stress, anxiety, depression, trauma, autism, and psychosis.

Social Bonding

Numerous studies have shown that singing in small and large groups increases social cohesion (Loersch & Arbuckle, 2013) and it appears that the larger the group, the greater the effect. There are also studies that reveal an increase in endorphin levels (neurochemicals akin to opioids), and increases in oxytocin as well, the neurochemical that underlies attachment. Endorphins are critical to increasing pain thresholds. Other studies have shown the release of dopamine, important in enhancing pleasure (Bostic et al., 2019; Chanda & Levitin, 2013).

Most recently, research has shown that the degree one is affected by listening to music is tied to one's sense of belonging to a group, and this likely has an evolutionary underpinning, related to group living. Thus, music helps us connect with groups (Clift et al., 2010). *After all, we humans are pack animals,* and affiliation with groups has long been a measure of survival. The combination of pleasure inducing neurochemicals, those that promote attachment, and the experience of affiliation and bonding, all enhance social connection and feelings of well-being.

In a pilot study researchers showed that when psychiatric patients, many suffering from psychosis, could jam with each other and with staff, both staff and the patients felt a greater sense of connection. Not only does this represent mutual recovery, but it also demonstrates that group cohesion is enhanced by "leveling the playing field," and all feeling part of a group. The jam group had a history of 9 years monthly and had no negative impact on treatment. Far from it. Many of the clinicians present in the jam sessions felt that their connection with patients improved and so did their treatment (Callahan et al., 2017).

Other research has revealed the value of singing in reinforcing mother–infant attachment. Maternal singing more than speech increased visual fixation, and decreased movement, indicating greater infant engagement. The researchers considered that the regularity and repetitiveness of singing (consider a lullaby), seemed to enhance attachment, compared with the variability of speech (Nakata & Trehub, 2004). Other studies have found that synchronicity, the matching of behavior and emotional states, was associated with better cognitive and behavioral development in infants. One way the mother relates to an infant through synchrony involves mutuality, reciprocity, rhythmicity, harmonious interaction, and turn taking through singing (Leciere et al., 2014).

Diminished Loneliness

Research by the British Broadcasting Corporation (BBC) and Cigna, in two large-scale studies, shows that the Gen Z and Millennials are the loneliest generation in the population, even more than the elderly (https://www.bbc.com/future/article/20180928-the-surprising-truth-about-lonliness, https://www.multivu.com/players/English/8294451-cigna-us-loneliness-survey/). The reasons for this are not clear, but the consequences are potentially significant. Loneliness has serious mental health consequences including emotional problems, such as increased risk for suicide; poor sleep and the consequences of sleep deprivation, including cognitive impairment, inattention, emotional blunting, and decreased productivity; difficulties with self-regulation evidenced by emotional over-eating, excessive drinking, smoking, substance misuse; and high cholesterol, increased blood pressure, and blunted immune response (Hawkley & Cacioppo, 2010).

While we don't know the reasons that young people are feeling so lonely, it is not as many people conclude, solely caused by overuse of social and digital media, but rather likely includes multiple causes such as over-scheduling and increased academic and other school pressures, community, and athletic related demands. It should be noted that these studies preceded the isolation due the pandemic but contributed to a perfect storm during it. To add to the storm, young people are worried and demoralized about the state of the world they are inheriting. Many are distressed about climate change, economic downturn, gun control, disparities against people of color, outright racism, marginalization of immigrants and LGBTQ young people, and sexual harassment among other social issues. These problems were often expressed by young people through groups and demonstrations, and then they faced the lockdown of COVID. A developmental derailment, and one that preceded COVID, with far too many issues to deal with noted above, as well as their own need for the normal developmental tasks of separation from family, autonomy, and identity formation, likely added to the perfect storm of loneliness and often attendant depression (Mushtaq et al., 2014). One study showed that loneliness had a significant impact on modulating negative emotions during lockdown (Chiu, 2020).

It should be noted that the second most common group sustaining loneliness are the elderly. Their situation is often compounded by loss, bereavement, and declining cognitive functioning. They too have associated depression along with their loneliness.

There are many ways to help, and one is the use of music. The two primary forms of musical intervention include active music therapy techniques, including singing, improvisation and music composition with lyric writing, and passive or receptive music therapy techniques, such as progressive muscle relaxation and guided imagery (Karapetsas & Laskarki, 2015). Some have pointed out that when improvising mirror neurons in the brain are activated, and when fired up, make us feel closer to others through the process of identification (Molnar-Szakacs & Overy, 2006).

Generally listening to music has been an effective means for mood regulation, expression of feelings and emotions, and this expression has been particularly robust in the elderly. Participation in group singing helps both young and old (Clift et al., 2010). Music creates a sense of social belonging when watching music videos with friends or sharing playlists. This is true for adolescents who simply listen alone or watch music videos or share playlists with friends. When listening, even when alone, the brain knows it came from a human agent, and hence is experienced as a social phenomenon. *When listening to music, you are never alone.*

Identity Formation

A key task for adolescents and young adults is in the formation of identity. This is a coherent sense of self, uniqueness from others, yet having the ability to affiliate with others in groups without losing one's personal qualities (Erikson, 1993). Ideally identity has continuity over time, and is often based on childhood memories, identification with important figures in life, yet differentiating oneself from them. It also often includes components, such as class, race, ethnicity, and spirituality. Healthy identity allows for modifications of one's values and ideals, coherent self-perception, increased awareness of how one compares oneself with others, and has a sound core that allows for an awareness of whether others perceive one accurately. This, of course, is no small task, and may be derailed by adverse childhood experiences that are traumatic. I among many other child and adolescent psychiatrists have considered this process of maturing, and solidifying identity extending beyond what we currently view as the "end" of adolescence (age 18), since the brain does not fully develop until about age 26.

The elements that enhance the formation of identity are many, and include the influence of parents and caregivers, childhood and teenage experiences including adverse childhood experiences and trauma, friends, mentors, spiritual and community leaders, and identification with others, the influence of social structures, including political, moral movements, and creative arts – books, movies, graphic art, theater, and music. Music is especially powerful, as it taps deeply into emotions, is inherently social, has agents with whom the young person identifies, and lyrics that may well help define their ideals, values, meaning and motivations in life (Miranda, 2013).

Music is deeply personal and is associated with seminal experiences in our lives, serving as a significant component of what we call autobiographical memories. Music has the ability at all stages of life to access what are considered self-defining periods (Loveday et al., 2020). Remember your first love? I am sure it was associated with songs that take you back to the emotions, connection, and power of that relationship. Remember other important times in your development – your experience in a social, athletic, or group event? This, too, was often associated with a song. Self-defining periods are not the sole province of music. They are also tied to books, films, athletic events, or family get-togethers. Music from the self-defining period is clearly significant to one's identity, and you know it because when you hear it you feel it deeply.

Adolescence is clearly when identity formation starts. It is a period of intense transformation as cognitive, biological, and social growth escalate. Erikson felt this was the time identity formation was initiated and suggested that teens needed a kind of psychosocial moratorium to process the wealth of concurrent forces impinging on them (Erikson, 1993). Sadly, today there is no time for a psychosocial moratorium – in fact, our youth are more barraged with duties, responsibilities, pressures, and a flood of input (much of which is digital) more than ever.

Despite the number of psychosocial stressors, most adolescents can adapt and meet the challenges they face. Music appears to be their soundtrack (see the reference to Dick Clark at the beginning of Chapter 1), and studies have found that they listen to music for an average of 2.5 hours a day (North et al., 2000). Music is a core building block of their identity, connecting them with peers and musical subcultures.

While many have assumed that music differentiates teens from their parents (and for most it does to some degree), the majority of adolescents generally adopt similar music preferences with their parents.

In fact, research in different cultures have shown that family listening to music together is extremely important in family cohesion (Boer & Abubakar, 2014). The same research demonstrated that music listening with peers is more important with their developmental stage and influence of the culture. What is most interesting is that many teens do not necessarily share identical musical preferences with their friends. Hence music provides a means for differentiation from parents and family; identification with parents; and a combination of shared and alternative music with friends. Sounds complex? It is! But consider that these are the variables that go into identity formation: unique preferences, shared and differentiated preferences with family; and how teens can have both common ground with those they hold dear, yet be unique in their tastes from their friends. All this is played out with musical choices.

How to adolescents use music? Many use music to find peace, emotional regulation, and validation. They also use music (and dance) to relieve tension and distract themselves from the complex challenges they face in life. It is key to coping with stress. There is interesting research on how music is used by girls versus boys. Whereas girls tend to use music for fulfilling their emotional needs, boys use music more for solidifying and showing off their social identity. Research shows that adolescents' emotional well-being is strongest when they have greater positive versus negative emotions from music and when they establish musical preferences with friends and family (Miranda, 2013).

Overall, music is extremely important to adolescent well-being. A large percent of teens are very involved with musical activities and have or do play an instrument. They prefer music to all other indoor activities with the possible exception of watching TV and use music for emotional regulation – to help them get through hard times, to relieve stress, to interact with friends, and to reduce loneliness.

There are situations when music will be used to support what Ericson called a negative identity. Some youth have considerable difficulty in navigation the waters of identity formation. In these cases, music and anti-heroes may champion a rejection of mainstream society, assail adult constraints and expectations, and survive alienation. This has been seen most vividly in metal or "shock rock." They were particularly known for their anti-establishment rituals and irreverence. They played with identity, embraced deeply uncomfortable issues such as death, mutilation and by doing so confronted unspeakable issues, and grappled gender identity in a very dramatic manner. (Bostic et al., 2003). These examples were flagrant demonstrations against their culture, the hypocrisy in society, and opposition to authority. For other teens, music may have a social, political, moral, and dramatic means of expressing themselves as separate from mainstream society.

While heavy metal focused on themes of alienation, mental confusion and hopelessness, and associated violence that seems to be self-directed, rap music and gangsta rap, in particular, appears instrumental in forming a community unified around race, inner-city life, standing up against oppression, and is geared toward socioeconomic and racial disparities (Reddick & Beresin, 2002).

In both of these cases, music does not serve to soothe emotions, but uses the emotional power of music to express themes of struggle and collective protest in a very blatant manner.

Regardless of the intentions, music plays a significant role in adolescent and young adult identity formation.

Peri-natal Emotional States

Research has demonstrated music to help in many situations involving procedures. We will see how it reduces anxiety, pre-and post-operatively. A large number of studies summarized by the WHO report (Fancourt & Finn, 2019) showing that music helps women in pregnancy, pre-labor, during labor and Cesarean sections, and after labor. For example, for women with pre-eclampsia, listening to music can reduce blood pressure and lower fetal heart rate (Cao et al., 2016). During pregnancy, listening to music is predictive of a better experience of labor, lower anxiety, decreased heart rate, increased fetal heart rate, shorter first-stage of labor, greater incidence of delivering naturally, and less need for medications (García González et al., 2018). During labor, listening to music lowers levels of anxiety, reduces pain, and leads to a faster progression of labor (Chuang et al., 2019). Finally, listening to music, increases positive emotions for women undergoing a Caesarean section along with lowering the need for pain meds, and reducing anxiety (Kushnir et al., 2012).

Improvement of Stress

We all experience stress, and though it is not a formal psychiatric diagnosis, there have been numerous studies looking at music and stress reduction. Background music is a great example. The exception to this finding is that many of us cringe at the background music when we are making calls and are put on hold. Steve Schlozman, a Boston physician, had such a negative reaction to the long waits and same music for years (and so did I!) that he complained to CVS, in a rather humorous letter published in the Boston NPR station newsletter *CommonHealth*. As physicians, we often must wait long periods of time to talk with pharmacists or to get approval for medications for our patients. The CVS music was the same for years and drove many of us over the edge. Steve complained in an elegant letter, and the music changed! But this is the exception to the rule. In this case background music increased stress (Schlozman, https://www.wbur.org/news/2018/05/25/cvs-hold-music).

In most cases, background music in public places is calming for most individuals. It is particularly helpful in reducing stress for those awaiting treatment (Cooke et al., 2005). This is often true in dental offices (Bare & Dundes, 2004). Background music may be particularly useful for children and the elderly awaiting and following surgical procedures.

In an experimental study, 60 women had salivary cortisol (the chemical released for the fight or flight response) along with heart rate, respiratory rate, and subjective stress perception when subjected to a psychological stress test(a simulation of a public speaking talk in applying for a job), and were broken into three groups subject to auditory stimulation before the stress test: one listening to relaxing music, a second listening to rippling water, and a third rest without any acoustic stimulation. The researchers found that listening to relaxing music prior to the stress test reduced the markers of stress with particular strong impact on heart rate, and perception of stress and to a lesser but positive degree, reduction in cortisol. This experimental situation demonstrated that music could modify the biological and perceptual components present in stress (Thoma et al., 2013).

Anxiety

Of all the psychiatric disorders, anxiety tops the list of conditions that are amenable to considerable reduction through music. We have seen above that anxiety is reduced in situations of pregnancy and labor. We have also noted that lullabies and maternal singing reduces anxiety and increases social bonding in infants (Nakata & Trehub, 2004). When music is played pre-operatively, patients have reported considerable reductions in anxiety, and similarly when music is played during procedures and post-operatively there is a significant reduction in anxiety. These situations are music in medicine techniques, in that music therapists are not used.

The robust response of anxiety reduction noted above involves clinical samples of subjects. Many of these studies were conducted using RCTs using varying measure of anxiety, such as cortisol levels, heart rate, blood pressure, respiratory rate, and measures (objective and subjective) of perceived anxiety.

What about the impact of music in reducing anxiety in non-clinical situations? One would think that if in situations high in stress, such as awaiting or following surgical procedures, music is highly effective in diminishing anxiety, it would be helpful in everyday life. One study looking at many RCTs found that listening to music revealed an overall decrease in self-reported anxiety. It was also effective for decreasing blood pressure, cortisol levels and heart rate, but the authors concluded that because of the great variability in the biological variables studied, they were cautious about concluding that it was effective in the biological arena (Panteleeva et al., 2017).

Depression

Depression is the number one burden of illness globally. It not only causes emotional distress, derails normal biological functioning such as sleep, appetite, and sexual functioning, impairs energy and concentration, reduces motivation and perhaps most concerning is that it is very closely linked to suicide. While medications and psychotherapy of various sorts are very effective (comparable compared to many other medical illnesses), there are several things outside traditional medical treatment that help improve depression – meditation, yoga, and some food supplements. But what about music? One could easily imagine that a lovely, moving, happy tune, perhaps associated with better times, would mitigate depression.

The bad news is that many researchers have noted that the data for music's reduction of depression are surprisingly lacking in strength, but the situation is not at all that clear to me. Many studies in adults and children have combined anxiety, depression, and other associated psychiatric disorders, and few did not venture away from using RCTs. We certainly need more studies that are qualitative and can look at depression apart from anxiety, stress, and other variables separately. Even more important would be to evaluate the role of music in depressed individuals, in terms of overall well-being.

In one large review of music interventions in treating depression, the authors noted that music interventions demonstrated a potential alternative for traditional therapy for depression, but the number of studies in current research literature is limited. These authors included both RCTs as well as longitudinal studies, and they differentiated passive listening and active singing, playing or improvising instruments. 1,810 subjects were included in their studies. They found that in 26 studies a statistically significant reduction in depression was found over time in the music intervention groups, particularly in elderly participants who showed robust improvement in depression whether listening or participating in music therapy projects. Group settings appeared to be more effective than solo cases. This makes sense. One of the fundamental principles for rising out of depression is the social support we receive from others (Leubner & Hinterberger, 2017).

In a study of nursing home residents with depression showed significant diminished depression following 2 weeks of music therapy. In the same study, analysis demonstrated greatly improved well-being in the nursing home residents who combined music with movement (Ray & Götell, 2018).

Trauma

Trauma can take on many forms. Post-Traumatic Stress Disorder (PTSD) is the most common and has three primary components: Remembering (such as flashbacks, vivid dreams, intrusive thoughts of the traumatic event); Emotional Numbing (evidenced by social withdrawal, reduced emotional response to others); and Arousal (basically, the fight or flight response including palpitations, hyper-ventilation, dizziness, nausea, feelings of impending doom – essentially a panic attack). I could see a role for music in each of these three domains. Music could distract from intrusive thoughts, and by association remind a person of positive, relaxing times. It could reduce emotional numbing, by group singing, dance, drum circles – ways of connecting with others through music (Carr et al., 2012). And finally, we have seen that music has a powerful calming effect on anxiety, and one can surmise that music might be able to reduce or even eliminate a panic attack.

Paradoxically, in my estimation, there is scant evidence that PTSD can be treated with music intervention. Some research with very small numbers shows that music interventions can decrease depression, increase pleasure, promote social bonding and com-munities, and facilitate emotional regulation. These studies must be considered preliminary, and future work is needed (Landis-Shack et al., 2017).

Since PTSD has significant components of arousal and anxiety, some researchers have begun to focus on dance and movement therapy. But the number of studies are small, and we await future work.

It seems to me that sadly we have many individuals who suffer from PTSD, particularly those who have served in the military, and first responders – police, fire fighters, EMTs and even Emergency Room clinicians. I hope that future research would target these vulnerable groups and initiate trials of music therapy.

Autistic Spectrum Disorder (ASD)

ASD is increasing in incidence and is for many a seriously debili-tating neurodevelopmental disorder with significant impairments in cognition, social communication, and behavioral functioning. It is not simply a serious disorder for children themselves, but has a huge emotional impact on parents, encompassing massive amounts of time, stress, and often financial hardship (paying for services, excessive time with the child and time away from work). The reason it is called a spectrum, is that there are some, who have normal intelligence, communication skills, an absence of behavioral abnormalities, and can become emotionally involved with others. Others are more severely affected, and those most severe require extensive time in rehabilitative units, outpatient programs along with home clinical care.

Some have argued that there are savants, who have ASD, and are musical geniuses, with the observation that a child may be severely affected by many of the debilitating features of ASD, who cannot communicate verbally, or socially, but can play the piano brilliantly, and by inference, that parts of the brain that may be preserved in ASD are amenable to music therapy.

While there are many models for treatment, largely through behavioral management and medications, there is considerable literature, largely case studies, that support the use of music therapy to improve communication, attention, and social connections, and to control stereotypic behavior in ASD. For example, during music therapy sessions, stereotypic behavior such as flapping decreased in some children.

While many researchers have been skeptical of the efficacy of music therapy in individuals with ASD, an extensive review of the literature including a wide range of studies, including randomized control studies among others as reported in the Cochrane Review (considered the gold standard of medical reviews), concluded that music therapy may help children with ASD to improve their skills in the primary areas of clinical difficulties in ASD: social interaction, verbal communication, social-emotional reciprocity, and initiating behavior. In addition, these studies support increasing social adaptation of kids and positive parent-child interactions (Geretsegger et al., 2014).

This is most promising, and even though it involved an extensive review, it only included 10 studies that met criteria for inclusion and 165 subjects. Clearly, we need more work in this area.

Psychosis

Of all psychiatric illnesses, the one that is often highly debilitating and most difficult to treat is the chronic psychotic disorder, schizophrenia. Those suffering from schizophrenia have what are classified as negative symptoms (withdrawal, lack of initiation, poor motivation, social isolation, depression), and positive symptoms (active delusions, hallucinations, paranoid thinking, aggressive behavior). Yet all psychosis is not schizophrenia. Bipolar disorder may have psychotic components that are a part of mania; and psychotic depression is a feature of this mood disorder. Fortunately, the mood disorders with psychosis are more amenable to treatment. But needless to say, they may be at times devastating and episodes require early intervention. While the cornerstones of treatment for psychosis is medication various forms of psychotherapy, music therapy may be instrumental in prevention and in various phases of intervention.

There have been few studies regarding the impact of music interventions with psychotic patients. However, in one meta-analysis while there was no difference between passive listening and structured music therapy groups, music was shown to be significantly effective in suppressing general symptoms of psychosis (Silverman, 2003). Other research has shown improvement in aggressiveness, paranoid thinking, hostility, and aggressiveness, as well as anxiety and depression (Volpe et al., 2018). In a Cochrane review, it was reported that music therapy in addition to standard care reduces general symptoms (hallucinations, delusions), social functioning, quality of life of people with schizophrenia. They note, however, that the data based on RCTs has low to moderate strength. Others have noted that music therapy in combination with standard treatment improved negative symptoms (social withdrawal, lack of motivation, poor social communication), as well as positive symptoms (delusions, hallucinations, hostility, and aggressiveness) (Tseng et al., 2016).

Thus, while there are only a few studies on psychosis, the positive impact on patients seems promising. I might add that the jam session noted above, in which many of the participants suffered from schizophrenia, also demonstrated an overall sense of well-being, social connectedness, initiation and positive communication.

B. PHYSICAL HEALTH

Music interventions have been incredibly successful in contributing to overall well-being and reducing symptoms in several medical conditions. These include dementia, stroke, Parkinson's disease, cardiac illness, and pain syndromes. It has also been effective in various settings including medical, surgical, nursing home and home-based settings.

Dementia

Dementia has many causes, but the most common is Alzheimer's Disease, a neurodegenerative illness that causes impairment in memory, finding the right words, visual and spatial orientation, disordered reasoning and judgment, and diminished attention and concentration. The behavioral component, include misplacing things, forgetting important tasks, such as turning off the stove, wandering and getting lost, and at times agitation and aggression. Many have emotional components, such as depression and anxiety. It is terribly painful for the individual in the early phases when they are acutely aware of losing functioning. And it is very painful for family members who remember their loved one as highly functional. Imagine your parent not recalling who you are. Many at moderate and certainly in later stages require assisted living, caregivers in the home, and at the end stages, memory units in nursing homes.

The focus on music interventions in dementia (and in most cases reviewed, Alzheimer's disease) are broad and have focused on the neuropsychiatric and behavioral symptoms as well as impaired cognition. In several studies music therapy improved disruptive behaviors, wandering, and anxiety levels. Music listening combined with reminiscence and attention training, along with physical exercise have demonstrated improved cognitive functioning, including executive functioning, orientation, and verbal expression (Sihvonen et al., 2017). Singing, listening and particularly group singing with rhythmic movements, and/or dance has been extremely effective in early dementia, with improvement in orientation, remote episodic memory, and autobiographical memory (Särkämö et al., 2014). Group singing has also improved interpersonal relationships and overall improvement in well-being (Osman et al., 2016). This may be one of the benefits of living in an assisted living situation or in a geriatric life center, where there is opportunity for group interaction, dancing, and music therapy.

Stroke

Stroke is an acute insult to the brain that may result from bleeding, for example from an aneurism or in a fall that causes bleeding in parts of the brain, or lack of oxygen to part of the brain, when, for example, one has a blood clot that blocks a blood vessel, or in severe cardiovascular illness when a blood vessel is narrowed significantly by atherosclerosis. Its clinical presentation may include any one of a number of symptoms, depending on the region of the brain affected. This could involve impaired speech (aphasia), motor or sensory abnormalities, diminished cognitive function such as short-term memory, attention and concentration, seizures, and more. Nonetheless, in the acute phase, it is terrifying, and often requires lengthy rehabilitation. It takes about 2 or more years for neurons to regenerate, and if the area is not significantly injured, there is hope for resumption of functioning. But only clinical evaluation and time will tell. Hence, the rehabilitation phase not only requires extensive physical and occupational therapy, but work on emotions, largely anxiety.

According to some researchers, the strongest evidence for the effectiveness of music-based interventions in medicine has been demonstrated for stroke (Sihvonen et al., 2017). Music therapy combined with dance have improved upper and lower limb functioning, muscular weakness, gait velocity, balance, and grip strength (Zhang et al., 2016). Music therapy has also resulted in decreased anxiety, depression, and overall improved well-being (Raglio et al., 2017). Singing has also shown to help stoke victims with aphasia (Simon, 2015).

Parkinson's Disease

Parkinson's disease is a neurodegenerative illness that is progressive and involves involuntary tremor, problems with gait, muscular stiffness, balance, coordination, speech, and mood disturbance.

It is slowly progressive and extremely distressing for the individual with the illness and for family who see progressive decline in functioning. The most consistent and effective musical treatment for Parkinson's Disease has been dance therapy, improving motor symptoms. Gait training using synchronized music improved velocity, stride, and cadence. Interestingly, the tango has been significantly more effective than waltz or foxtrot (Hackney & Earhart, 2009). In some studies, combining singing with walking was effective in cuing gait (Sihvonen et al., 2017).

Cardiac Illness

The two most common cardiac illnesses are coronary artery disease, associated with heart attacks, and arrhythmias. These disorders are often associated with significant anxiety and are very responsive to surgical intervention for placement of arterial stents or bypass procedures, for coronary artery disease and medication management for arrythmias. In both conditions, cardiologists worry about blood pressure, and heart rate. These disorders cause significant anxiety that may be dangerous if arousal is increased. Multiple studies have reported that music can significantly reduce anxiety in patients with heart disease. Furthermore, music therapy has demonstrated reduction in pain, though the effect is small to moderate. Additional music interventions may lower blood pressure, heart rate and respiratory rate (Koelsch & Jancke, 2015). Interestingly, and I think importantly, the most profound effects of music on the heart are by improving mood and anxiety. Emotional factors, including stress, are powerful contributors to heart disease and rehabilitation from heart attacks (Bradt et al., 2013).

Pain Syndromes

Many illnesses, accidents, and procedures cause pain. We have all lived with pain, and each of us have thresholds for pain, some lower and some higher. The quick fix for pain is to reach for non-steroidal anti-inflammatory medications (such as ibuprofen, naproxen) but these run the risk of gastrointestinal bleeding. Others turn to opioids and run the risk of addiction. There are several non-medical adjunctive treatments for pain, such as meditation, yoga, and acupuncture. Music can substantially diminish pain through passive listening, music therapy, and in community music production (Bernatzky et al., 2012). While the mechanism may be the production of endorphins or opioids, reduction in anxiety, a known contributor to the experience of pain, distraction, or the relevance of social supports, we know that it works. And, importantly, it works on virtually every source of pain. In my experience, when we combine music interventions, with other forms of treatment that reduce pain, such as meditation, conventional medications, physical and occupational therapy, cognitive-behavioral and other forms of psychotherapy, the combination of interventions summate. The range of disorders producing pain is extensive from migraine to fibromyalgia (Linnemann et al., 2015) and many other conditions that produce some of the most intense pain. And we have seen that music interventions helps with pain during labor and delivery.

The Use of Music in Medical and Home Care Settings

While there is considerable heterogeneity of disorders treated in medical, surgical, and consultation services (Rafieyan & Ries, 2007), assisted living facilities, nursing homes, and in home-based care (Schmid & Ostermann, 2010), there are a wealth of studies to show that the addition of music, passive or active music therapy can be an invaluable adjunct to the way we care for patients and each other. All benefit from music in these settings.

While we are all aware of the limitations of adding to the already skyrocketing costs of healthcare, the addition of music, even passive music would not add much to our overhead, and in fact, if it could decrease the needs of patients for staff time through relaxation, we may even be able to afford music therapists in these settings through significant cost savings. The bottom line is that if we think creatively, we can incorporate a low cost and effective modality to our services and all benefit.

3

WHO BENEFITS? STORIES OF MUSIC ENHANCING PERSONAL AND PROFESSIONAL WELL-BEING

VIGNETTES: A BRIEF INTRODUCTION

In Chapter 1, we described health as embracing well-being, and clarified well-being as having a number of components, as indicated by PERMA +4, including Positive Emotions, Engagement, Meaning, and Accomplishments. We also noted that Seligman added 4 components we should include in our appraisal of well-being: Physical Health, Mindset (and in particular, a growth mindset), Workplace, and Financial Security.

I pointed out that not everyone has all components nor is well-being linear. After all, one can have a serious, even fatal illness and overall maintain positive well-being. And well-being is not based on our being happy all the time. We get thrown off every so often. It is a matter of being resilient, flexible, and maintaining a "tool kit" of coping mechanisms to get us back on track. One tool is the personal use of music.

In this chapter, the heart of this book, there are several deeply personal vignettes. These narratives convey the broad scope and use of music personally and professionally and are written by a heterogeneous group of people – from a former patient of mine to friends, clinicians, and music therapists. In some cases, I will add an introduction if the situation merits clarification, such as the one contributor who is a former patient. Others stand on their own.

VIGNETTES

I Can Do This All Day

The view of the nameplate outside the door lets you know something about what's coming before you ever set foot into my office. The Fender Telecaster magnet, in a beautiful sunburst finish, sits quietly at an angle just below my name. Ever since I can remember, I just couldn't get enough of guitars.

It doesn't matter how old it is, or how damaged it may appear; I think an angel must get its wings each time I set eyes on a guitar. I've been drawn to them ever since I first became aware of the Beatles at age five and saw John Lennon playing his iconic Rickenbacker 325 on the cover of *Something New*. How many times did I take tracing paper to that cover to draw, and then redraw, that solid black, tulip-shaped guitar? Upon entering my office, you can see that guitar in Lennon's hands in November of 1960 as he sits atop a truck in Hamburg in a black and white photo taken by Astrid Kirchherr, the woman who originated the Beatles' mop-top haircuts.

Turn right through the door of my office, behind the consultation area where I do my clinical work, and you'll see my "studio" – in and amongst the baskets of toys and blocks and surrounded by bookshelves on three sides stand a brilliant orange Gretsch Chet Atkin's semi-hollow body, a honey burst Fender Stratocaster, and a 4-watt, creamy red, hand wired Vox amp. Once upon a time, I brought them into the office for my teenage patients; to help them loosen up, speak more easily, play a bit, and see me as relatable. It took me a year or two to realize that, in fact, while they still serve that purpose, I actually brought them in for me.

Some days, I just glance at the guitars briefly, comforted by their presence, shielding me in some respects from the despair of my patients, and the disappointment and fears of their parents. But most days, in between the hours spent with patients, the far too many administrative fires that require extinguishing, and the joyful care and watering of students and trainees, I turn to my guitars for 5 or 10 minutes of rejuvenation and unadulterated pleasure.

The guitars sit within arm's reach of my desk chair. I swivel, I grab, and I give the guitar a single strum. Are we in tune? Close enough for rock 'n' roll, and I'm off. I'll sharpen or flatten as needed from here.

Sometimes I play a series of riffs. Sometimes I get back to something I'm working on, a song or solo, but most often I improvise. I find myself moving unreservedly around the neck, building melodies off chords, and finding my way back home. While almost everyone who enters my office comments on the guitars, it surprises me still that only the minorities want to wrap their hands around these six-stringed pieces of wood and metal and give it a go. It surprises me because they matter so deeply to me. For me, the guitar emotes, transforms, calms, and provides immense joy. These positive feelings are important for me to be reminded of throughout my day.

Occasionally, if the mood hits me, and my office door is shut, I might even sing a bit. It feels good. In the midst of an unknowing and impossible day, I feel competent and in control.

Sometimes I think I missed my calling. Maybe, if I had the right training and encouragement, or if I wasn't so interested in learning and medicine and social justice, I would have been a professional musician. Maybe. But I'm not convinced I have the chops. I tell myself that when I retire, I'll spend my nights playing blues in bars. Another maybe. For now, 10 minutes here and there will have to do. Guitar playing gives me a place to reflect and recharge. A guitar in my hands is akin to Captain America's shield in his. Like the Captain says, "I can do this all day."

Jess P. Shatkin, MD, MPH
Professor of Child & Adolescent Psychiatry and Pediatrics
NYU Grossman School of Medicine

Music and Me

When I was in high school, every weekend, I'd walk 20 minutes out of my neighborhood to the nearby nursing home. I would sign in at the front desk, then amble over to the upright piano in the corner of their large eating area. After a couple tries, I learned that if I went around dinner time, most of the residents would be in this common space.

Here, I would play for about an hour every night. I played a mix of classical and hymnal music, as well as any requests I had gotten from the residents. At first, it was incredibly awkward, as I was barely 15 years old, in front of 50 or so strangers. But over the years, I learned to forget the age difference, and the unfamiliarity of it all. We could simply connect through the notes emanating from the piano, and in those hours, music was our only language.

There is something uniquely healing about music. The rhythm, the melody, the harmony, each and every aspect of a musical piece does something to the mind and soul. Ever since I was a little kid, whenever I'd get my usual recurrent migraine, sitting in front of the piano and just playing for even 30 minutes would cause the throbbing pain to dissipate. When playing for other people, it was extraordinary to notice how starting a piece on the piano would cause silence to fall over any room. It was trancelike, as if time had frozen and the melody itself was dictating the flow of everyday life.

When I play or listen, there is simultaneously something soothing yet exhilarating, as if I am saying goodbye with every hello. There is a story, one alive and full of feeling, in every note and phrase. Much like the written word, music provides a template to translate thoughts and emotions. But unlike our written word, music is universally understood without any prior training. People just *know* when a piece is sad or hopeful, uplifting or angry. It continually reminds me of our shared humanity and consciousness.

I first started playing around age 5. There was an old piano in the half-furnished apartment we just moved into. Having recently immigrated from China, we had little to nothing, with no knowledge of American language or culture. But as the ever-curious child, one day I opened the piano lid and banged on a couple keys. My parents interpreted that as an interest in music and took me to my first piano teacher. I don't remember the story, but apparently, she took one look at my hands and declared I was unteachable, since my hands were too small. And as I grew up and became her star student, she would still unabashedly tell this story to all her students, with a loud hearty laugh.

To me, music has always been an endless supply of raw feeling, the continual making of *something* out of *nothing* That is why ever since I was young, I loved playing Chopin, with all his rubato and storytelling. Each of his pieces was so incredibly malleable, as if he provided you with the brush and paint, and the canvas was for you to draw. I also think that feeling of unfiltered, unprocessed *creation* was what made music so exciting. It was you, an instrument, and a score to follow. Nothing more, nothing less.

In college, I realized that this love and thrill for music could be shared in more intentional ways. I joined a music club my freshman year, playing music at nursing homes every week with a team of classmates. We'd host mini-concerts, but also mingle with the residents afterwards. It reminded me of high school, but this time, the intentionality was different. Back then, I was playing for the sake of playing. Now, I realized that the pieces I chose, the conversations I would have, could not only serve as artifacts of art, but vessels for connection and empathy. As a poet as well, I wrote about the power music and poetry had both in my life and the medical profession for my medical school personal statement, and at every interview, every person I spoke with always agreed with me.

In medical school, I've also sought ways to share music with patients. As a student without much else to offer, music is one way to channel any healing I can provide. And even if brief, I've noticed that music is truly healing. It stirs something in you, leaves you wondering how broken and beautiful we all are. There is a steadfast inspiration in that thought for me, while also deeply comforting.

Music has always and will continue to be deeply restorative for me. When I experienced the loss of a loved one last year, closure for me was not achieved in saying goodbye or writing reflections about it. Rather, it was sitting at the piano and playing a piece that reminded me of her. When my life feels tumultuous and uncertain, music has been the perpetual anchor of my mind, providing both an escape and a way forward. I know music will forever be a source of healing and hope. It is impossible to put into words exactly what my relationship with music has been like, but then again, I don't think there exists a perfect label for that. Instead, it would be better understood if I played a piece and shared some music with you.

David Xiang
Harvard Medical Student

Into the Darkness We Will Ride

The tide that never ceases to ebb and flow;
The flame that resists the blow.
Words and sounds, blood and sweat,
Love and pain, joy and regret.
You connect us all and define the times
With deafening amps and poignant rhymes.
What would I be without you?
A lifeless portrait of absent hue.
The work I do is empathy;
Emotional connectivity.
Show me the way to the inside;
I'll follow the steps you deftly guide.
To hearts and minds, a map to souls,
Helping me navigate these rocks and rolls.
The syllabus to the human form,
Constantly reminding me there is no norm.
Comfort my soul when I am down.
Guide my ship into your sound.
Provide the light for dazzling eyes,
Shimmering notes that endlessly rise.
Fight with me as I scream with rage,
A wild beast without a cage.
Pace my heart to the beat of love,
Aching rain down from above.
Can I ever repay you for what you've done?
Compensate you for wars you've won?
Accept this ode as my tithe
For keeping my dreaming tree alive.
I will forever call you friend,
Mother, father, my closest kin

And when I take my final sigh,
Music, into the darkness we will ride.

John Tyson, MD
Instructor in Psychiatry, Harvard Medical School
Attending, First Episode Psychosis Program
Singer, Songwriter, Guitarist for Gideon Grey

Personal Vignette on Music and Medicine

Without even realizing what I was doing, I pushed open the door advertising "Most Patient Teachers in Town" and signed up for bass lessons. I was on my Surgery rotation, the coldest, bleakest point of my 3rd year of medical school, and I passed the John Payne Music Center every day as I walked to the hospital in the predawn darkness. I'd been playing the bass since I was 8 years old, with more enthusiasm than expertise, and my "chops" (playing ability) were stagnant. I didn't have extra time or money, but I walked in anyway; those lessons pushed me up to a whole new level of jazz playing and pushed me on through the rest of 3rd year.

Far from being just a hobby, music has been integral to my career as a pediatrician, albeit indirectly. I enjoy playing in rock and jazz bands at parties, clubs, and art galleries, singing and writing songs. It's fun but also energizing, not so much for relaxation as for rejuvenation. Music is one of the essentials that keep me engaged in my work and prevent burnout.

I'm fond of incorporating music into teaching and research activities. I've used my rudimentary guitar playing skills to accompany myself on "singing lectures" for medical students and residents on topics ranging from encopresis to Attention-Deficit/Hyperactivity Disorder to the common cold; for orientation presentations to groups of students; and for study jingles and recruitment of colleagues in a national pediatric practice-based research network. Music wakes up the audience and helps them remember the message.

Although I don't sing or play music in my office where I spend the lion's share of my time, I am always mindful of the parallels between jazz bass playing and primary care pediatrics. The bass has an important supportive, accompanying role in most bands; as a pediatrician I support children and families and accompany them from birth into early adulthood. The great bass player Ray Brown, in the liner notes to his album of duets with Duke Ellington, wrote that more than playing fast or soloing, it's important that a bass player "just lays down some good time, with a good sound and good intonation." I strive for this goal when I play the bass, and I strive for it as a pediatrician. My colleagues who are cardiologists and oncologists and neurosurgeons perform jaw-dropping feats of care for serious illnesses; they are the flashy players. But for me as a primary care pediatrician to have good time, I need to figure out when to intervene and when to reassure, when a child's development is delayed and when she is simply following her own trajectory, when another child's symptoms require laboratory testing and medications and when he needs lifestyle counseling and "tincture of time." And to have a good sound and intonation, I need to find the right words and tone of voice to establish and maintain a therapeutic alliance with each child and family–to ask the right questions, give clear explanations, and offer appropriate guidance.

I don't play the bass while I'm seeing patients, but Ray Brown's words stay with me in the exam room. Playing (and listening to) music are uplifting, nourishing, and sustaining to me personally and professionally, as the late rock critic Lester Bangs put it, "because the best music is strong and guides and cleanses and is life itself."

Benjamin Scheindlin, MD
Assistant Professor of Pediatrics Part-Time
Harvard Medical School

A Mostly True Story

48 1/2 years ago, ~Feb 14 a 24-year-old white kid who recently lost 20 lbs down to ~125 after 2 weeks of no eat/no sleep psychosis with full beard not well groomed and hair half way down his back, looking and sounding more like an Old Testament prophet than anything else trying to not be a fifth horseman of the Apocalypse; a nuclear device. He's been heavily medicated and let out of seclusion for the first time and into the Day Room where several other patients are scattered around not talking, in their own worlds. There's an old upright piano which I walk up to tentatively checking the tuning which is not good but could be worse. I start playing chords from the songs in BRINGING IT ALL BACK HOME, some

patients walk over and then we begin to sing the words. In ten minutes or so we have our own version of three part harmony. One of the patients says that I play well.

"Not really but I'll be back."

To this day, I wouldn't dream of living without a piano and I have one in the office in the art room which my patients can play with and sometimes I play with them.

Mark Vonnegut, MD

Primary Care Pediatrician

Author

On Music, Communication and Mental Health

As a psychiatrist, I am fascinated by the connection between music and mental health. Music does not come up with every patient, but for some, it can play a major role. My first psychotherapy patient in residency was a man in his 60s who had suffered extensive emotional trauma in childhood and had lived an extremely isolated life ever since. For him, outside of psychotherapy (which he faithfully attended), the music of Bob Dylan was one of his sole companions and sources of connection to other humans. I recall a woman in her early 20s with borderline personality disorder who shared with me the original music that she composed and performed. The recordings conveyed her inner experience of angst, vulnerability, and longing in a way that surpassed what she could communicate through spoken words alone. Another patient was a banker with two children in his late 30s, whose memory of childhood was cold and emotionless. I was surprised when he told me that one of the few things that induced strong feelings in him was musical theater. The combination of harmony and lyrics, he explained, touched him in a way very few other experiences could. For all these individuals, music offered a means of communication, a way in, a bridge.

I am also an amateur violinist. At different times in my life, music has played all these roles for me as well – a comfort, a catharsis, and a means of conveying inner emotion. For a while I had the great pleasure of playing in a classical string quartet with colleagues including a psychologist-cellist, a psychiatrist-violist, and a neuroscientist-violinist. We called ourselves "Folie a Quatre," a play on a psychiatric syndrome describing a shared delusion. Together, we explored the music of composers who were thought to have suffered from mental illness and speculated as to what might be communicated through the notes on the page. In the first movement of Robert Schumann's Quartet No. 3 in A Major, for example, we found ourselves plagued by a devilishly challenging syncopated rhythm undergirding an otherwise sunny and lyrical passage; the net result, we all agreed, was that we felt ill-at-ease and off-kilter. Schumann suffered bouts of what today would likely be described as depression and mania, and he ended his days in an asylum following a suicide attempt. Many evenings were spent speculating whether Schumann was using music to express an inner experience, whether musical creation occurred because of or in spite of mental illness, and how music might promote healing in our patients. I am certain that music has affected my understanding of humanity as well as my practice of psychiatry.

Justin Chen, MD, MPH

Medical Director Outpatient Psychiatry Division

Massachusetts General Hospital

Assistant Professor, Harvard Medical School

My Guitar

Looking back now at more than 40 years of practicing psychiatry, I have been touched by how hard life can be, how unfair and full of misery for many people. I've also come to appreciate the value of human kindness and the power of warm human relationships, from nurses, counselors, doctors, and others, in offering succor, support and fellowship as balms for suffering. I've come to see the human family as capable of great kindness and mutuality, and that this capacity for lovingkindness is deeply redemptive – for both the carer and the recipient of care. Over the years I've also come to realize how varied, and sometimes surprising, are the pathways to recovery, health and fulfillment.

Music – and especially music made with friends – has exemplified for me this life-affirming spirit, and springboard to well-being. I am a decidedly mediocre, but very enthusiastic, music maker. Still, music and my beloved guitar have been great gifts in my life.

About 10 years ago, I had the amazing experience of building my own guitar. I'd like to say it was built by my hands, and to a degree it was, but I was guided, overseen, and rescued so frequently by my luthier/guitar teacher and dear friend, Arthur Olins, that it is more accurate to say that it was built mainly by him, with secondary help from me.

Arthur builds guitars and teaches guitar building in his basement workshop, where he offers a class on Monday nights. Students pay a shop fee and then build guitars under Arthur's supervision. The workshop also has a pool table, a big screen TV, and a refrigerator, which students are expected to stock with beer as part of their shop fees. Accordingly, the pace of building guitars is very, very slow. The whole place has the feel of an 11-year-old's boys club, complete with fart jokes, baseball games on the TV, and general raunchiness. In other words, it's heaven.

I met Arthur about 30 years ago. It started on a whim. I was driving along and passed a music store that offered lessons in its window. I'd plunked along on a guitar for years, basically playing the same three chords, strumming haphazardly, entirely for my own amusement. When I saw the lessons sign, a seed of an idea appeared: why don't I actually learn to play the guitar? I thought: it's a choice. This is my one precious life – why not go for it?

So, I found my way back to the store, went in, and arranged for some lessons. I showed up for my first one and was introduced to Arthur, who led me up a narrow staircase to his tiny studio, and we began, with Arthur showing me the proper way to hold the guitar and introducing me to basic chords and their structure. From the start I was a lousy student. Despite my commitments to the contrary, I hardly practiced, and when things didn't come quickly, I didn't persist. Arthur hung in there with me, but he seemed to lose interest in my lessons – no doubt because I was showing up not having practiced. In any case, he had a habit of gazing out the window, seeming bored. It was here that I almost made a critical mistake that could have changed the course of my life: I asked the store proprietor if there were any other guitar teachers available. Thank god, he said no, and assured me that Arthur was an excellent teacher. Had I actually changed teachers, I'd have missed out on one of the great friends, and great gifts, of my life.

My guitar's top is spruce. For the back and sides of the guitar, Arthur had the very last remains of a board of Brazilian rosewood that he'd taken in trade for some guitar repairs about 20 years before. The rosewood is a rich, dark, deep coffee brown, lustrous and warm. The neck is mahogany, and the fingerboard is ebony – a flat, midnight black. The sound hole is ringed with a circle of abalone shell, and the outline of the guitar top is similarly bordered by a line of abalone – a gorgeous, luscious, multicolored shell, that shimmers kaleidoscopically in any light. A twisting vine of abalone also runs up the fingerboard, and into the headstock, among the tuning pegs. I'd found this dazzling vine on a website: a Vietnam war veteran had returned to Vietnam after the war and founded a factory in which these inlays are built by hand. All in all, the guitar is a marvel, just this side of gaudy, or maybe a bit on the other side of gaudy.

My guitar deserves a much better player. When Arthur plays my guitar, it sounds magnificent – full and rich, and capable of anything. I really can't begin to do it justice. But like a proud father of a child whose accomplishments astonish her parents, I take a great deal of joy in being connected with this beautiful instrument.

About 20 years ago, through another piece of amazing serendipity, my wife Julie and I were introduced to neighbors, Carol and Jeff, who lived around the corner from us and we discovered that we all liked to play music. We got together a couple of times and played folk tunes and some rock and roll, lubricated by some adult beverages. We had a great time. It turned out that Carol and Jeff had some other friends and we had some friends, and before you knew it, we had a monthly music-making group, rotating from house to house, with pot luck dinners contributed by everyone. It turned out to be absolutely wonderful. We've been meeting at least monthly ever since.

Ten years after that, I got the idea that a monthly music jam could be a very cool idea for the company where I work –a non-profit, social service agency that provides all sorts of services for people who are experiencing psychiatric conditions, developmental and other cognitive challenges, substance use conditions and other life difficulties, all with the goal of promoting rewarding self-directed lives. A colleague there, Alan Crane, was a wonderful guitar player, and he and I gathered a few other people and decided to start a Monthly Music Jam.

Initially, our idea was to rent a church hall, and put on a music jam for people to come listen and sing along. We put together song books, took requests, and served pizza. Lots of people came, and everyone seemed to love it. But almost immediately, it transformed into a much more communal, participatory experience. People didn't want to just be sung to, *they wanted to make music themselves*. So it rapidly shifted to being more of an open mike, with people singing, playing instruments, tap dancing, singing acapella, telling stories, reading poems, sometimes with the help of the "house band" led by Alan Crane, and sometimes without. It was a joyous, riotous noise. The skill level of the participants varied a lot but the atmosphere was 100% supportive and encouraging. It was life lived large.

I've been a life-long worrier, prone to brooding and catastrophizing, and susceptible to horrifying panic attacks, all of which have been substantially helped – though not eliminated – by various kinds of psychotherapy and psychiatric medications. I am very good at talking myself into being anxious. But one place I am pretty much entirely at ease is when we are making music. Playing with friends helps me remember that life can be good, that the human family can be warm, accepting, supportive, and merry-making. And the music itself, clunky or magnificent, reminds me that there is a quality of reality that is truly worthy of reverence. Beside all that, music is also a magical way out of the rabbit hole of pathological self-consciousness – back to the world of rhythm and well-being.

Making music is a great example of an idea that psychiatrists have long embraced: life does the healing. Most of our work is to help people get involved in the great, wild project of being alive, and not imprisoned in the sterile world of isolated, often harshly critical, self-absorption.

Chris Gordon, MD
Chief Medical Officer, Emeritus, Advocates, Inc
Associate Professor, part time, Harvard Medical School

Music Through My "Ages and Stages"

I don't think I knew just how important music was to me until it wasn't there. Growing up, I played the violin and the piano; my parents were always listening to music at home. In 9th grade, my family and I moved to another state, and my new high school had no orchestra! I met with the band director, and he started me on the

French horn. I wasn't great, but I kept at it and loved it, motivated to get better so that I could eventually join the marching band and wind ensemble. Being in the marching band with all my friends at football games, parades, and competitions was truly the highlight of my high school existence.

When I started college at University of Delaware, I thought for sure I would join the marching band. But I feared I wasn't good enough, and I was overwhelmed with homesickness, academic challenges, and meeting new people, so I stopped after one practice. As freshman year continued, and as I struggled to navigate college life and figure out a routine and study strategy that worked for me, I experienced a heavy feeling that something was missing. That summer, I recuperated at home, spending time with my family and friends. By the time I returned for sophomore year, it had finally dawned on me that it was music missing from my life! I talked to someone in the music department and began taking French horn lessons for credit; I also joined the symphonic band during my junior year. It was actually exhilarating to trudge over to the music building, even on cold evenings, to practice. Being there made me feel like I was part of something special, all of us doing something we loved: making music. I remember the sense of accomplishment at having realized that something was missing, figuring out what it was, and doing something to fill that emptiness and balance me. From then on, I made every effort to keep music integrated into my life however possible.

After college, I moved to NY for graduate school, bringing my keyboard and a few music books for my apartment. I discovered an *a cappella* group and began singing. I loved discovering my voice and enjoyed directing the group during my last two years of graduate school. Then I went to medical school, where there didn't seem to be much time for anything besides studying (and going into Manhattan on weekends). However, I began working at the Student Center a few evenings a week and discovered Dessert Night, where the co-founders of Music That Heals, a program that brings music to people in hospitals and other healthcare facilities, would play guitar and sing while I served cheesecake to students in the audience. One night, the ladies must have noticed me singing along to myself and asked me to join them. From then on, they would invite me to sing a few songs with them every Dessert Night. Sing-ing with them gave me something to look forward to and broke up the "seriousness" of medical school. I still send them Christmas cards and donate to Music That Heals to this day.

After Psychiatry residency and Child and Adolescent Psychiatry fellowship, I moved to Michigan for my first job. I promised myself I would fulfill my dream of joining a community choir as an official "grown-up" with a job and a house. I found one in town, tried out, and began singing with the Livingston County Women's Choir. It was great fun. I loved the practices and all the wonderful women I got to know there. Many of them were a few decades older than I and had been singing for years. They took me under their wings and became a sort of surrogate family, as my husband and I had no family nearby. They rejoiced when I got pregnant and threw me baby showers before each of my children were born. I still send some of them Christmas cards every year.

In the early years of motherhood, my children were the focus of everything I did (other than go to work part-time). We took walks, explored new places, spent a lot of time at the library. Every night, I read and sang to them before bed so that they, too, would grow up with music and literature. When my daughter was 5 years old, she started playing the violin. Her tiny 1/10th size violin was so cute! Sometimes she needed me to play a short duet with her, so I had to break out the violin my parents had given me so long ago! After a hiatus of 30 years, it was amazing to feel the music flow back into my fingertips. I will admit that I did not anticipate the delight I would feel at playing again.

Now here I am, having come full circle to the very first instru-ment I ever played, a few instruments (including my voice!), four degrees, two kids, multiple relocations, and several years later! I look forward to my lessons, and it's something I do just for me. However, when I spend extra time on the tough parts of various pieces, I like to think that my children are also learning something. As they hear me make mistakes and play the same thing over and over again, they see a live example of how things don't come eas-ily, even to "grown-ups": you have to try hard and practice to get better at anything.

Through my life, I've come to the realization (many times) that music is truly a gift. It makes me happy; it has brought me together with people I would not have otherwise known; it keeps my brain active; it teaches life lessons. Just hearing a few notes of a song can evoke powerful memories of what I was doing, where, and with whom when that song was playing. It brings me joy to think what an ever-present role music has had in my life and makes me so grateful for the opportunities that I have had to engage in it myself and with others that are important to me and to share it with my children.

Liwei L. Hua, MD, PhD
Integrated Child and Adolescent Psychiatrist
South Bend Clinic
South Bend, IN

Be With Me Music

E-E-E-E-D-D-A-A... E-E-E-E-D-D-A-A...with staccato gusto I bang out the chords on my Silvertone guitar as our band of 8th graders belts out "And her name is G—L—O—R—I—I—I... G-L-O-R-I-A.... Gloria!" And it is Glorious. I still smile as I remember the exuberance, the joy, the thrill of making this music together. My mother somehow allowed our band, the Next of Kin, to rehearse in our family's den and as I think back it brought a smile to her face. And it was loud, which added to the raucous joy of it all. Maybe what I am describing is the sense of freedom this brought to my conventional suburban life. But it was more than that. It was a way to communicate. A way to connect with and express myself. A way to connect with others. A way to connect to the past and the future. Our bass player was Ron T and he sounded just like James Taylor when he sang. Ron and I would listen to Beatles albums for hours in his bedroom marveling at every nuance in their voices, harmonies, and ensemble playing. Ron and I have remained close friends throughout our lives. Through every chapter of life almost all of my closest friends are people that I have played music with. The hours playing music with Jay H, Gene, Tony, and the other members of Pink Freud, along with the hours of relaxing, sipping whiskey, letting our guards down, talking honestly, and serving as guideposts for living have been foundations of my life. One of my mentors in residency, Carl Whitaker, used to say that to survive adult life we all need a "cuddle group." My cuddle group has been the friends I have played music with.

Words can be deceptive but music is authentic, connects directly to the Limbic System as George Murray wrote about. No forked tongues in music. It was one of the few nonconflictual spheres I could enjoy with both my parents. It was and remains a joyous way I connect with our children. I have written songs for each of the new members of our family and when our first grandson (Alex Bernard, named after his great grandparents on each side) was born last year the song I wrote threaded together past, present, and future with the words:

W-W-W-Welcome sweet Alex

Your middle name is Bernard

The whole world really needs you

To clean up this mess of a yard

Music has brought comfort, solace, deep connections with others, and given me a way to articulate what is hard to express verbally. The map is not the territory and words capture only some of our experience. I often resonate with particular pieces of music and recognize "Yes that's exactly how I feel!" In this way, music provides hope that we can be understood, that we can be heard, that others feel the same way, that we are not alone in the world. This is a powerful message that is even more pressing today in our changing-at-warp-speed, COVID-tinged world. Music is a connector that can potentially bridge the worrisome fault lines that have emerged in the past decade. Music permeates all I do with patients, friends, and family.

One of my favorite painters is the late Catherine Burchfield Parker, one of whose last paintings was entitled *Be With Me Music*, inspired by the poem of the same name by Augustine Towey. The painting is a triptych of the progression of the day from morning until night, with the sounds of music in evidence all the while until the end of the day. It reminds me of a quote by Bruce Springsteen: *"The best music is essentially there to provide you something to face the world with"*.

Whatever comes may music be with us.

David Kaye, MD
Vice-Chair of Academic Affairs, Psychiatry
Jacobs School of Medicine and Biological Sciences
University of Buffalo Department of Psychiatry
Professor of Psychiatry, University of Buffalo
Band member, Pink Freud and the Transitional Objects

Music in an After-School Program

The MGH Revere Youth Zone is an after-school and summer program in which I've been involved since I was old enough to be a member myself. I have seen the program grow and change over the years, watching as waves of timid new faces turn to smiles as they find their place, and eventually graduate from the program with the rest of their lives stretching far out in front of them.

The change that I have found most impressive – perhaps due to my own predilections – has been the integration of music into the Youth Zone (the YZ, as we call it). Sparing the details of how music became woven into the daily doings at the YZ, members now have opportunities to learn to play instruments, participate in a music history and technology club, and perform choreographed dances with their friends through a fan-favorite video game. These activities give members the chance to be creative, developing their musical skills and knowledge in a safe and fun space along with their friends and classmates. Music has become an outlet through which the kids can express, communicate, and build bonds by teaching and learning the language of music together.

There is certainly much to gain from the music at the YZ, but there is one thing the kids always seem to lose: their inhibitions. The socially guarded older kids will use emotional language to describe how a song sounds; how it makes them feel. The quiet student will test her knowledge and skills on the guitar so she can teach the tidbits she knows to a starry-eyed newcomer. Exclusive cliques of teens who are just too cool for school will heckle their friends' moves while they wait in unspoken anticipation for their turn to join the ragtag dance crew themselves.

This is how music breaks barriers.

Adolescent social life is turbulent, to put it lightly. It's riddled with all the trappings of your favorite soap opera. Betrayal, injustice, love, and loss, seething hatred, distrust, and the always-lingering sense of confusion. This is the formula for an average day at an average school for the average 8th grader. But just like in the TV dramas, there is always a way out.

Like the reveal of the protagonists' evil twin as the cause of all the suffering, music lets us see things – see each other – in a new light, and a fresh perspective is a scarce resource for most young folks. Caught up between studying, extracurriculars, and trying to fit it in, life in middle and high school is a landslide of questions with very few answers. But when we start digging into music, those answers seem to lose their weight.

This is how music brings solace.

A much-needed reprieve from the pageantry of being cool in the classroom, music is a great equalizer. We all find ourselves on a level playing field when music takes the stage. Your answer is as good as mine. The chords, the scales, the dance moves, the favorite (and most despised) songs and singers make up the alphabet of a language that anyone, anywhere, at any time can speak.

This is what music means to me, and this is how music causes togetherness. When you like a song, you dance or sing along. Or maybe you cry. Your connection to a tune will always be yours, but it can also be a story to share, a reason to speak your mind, a way to hear more clearly the voices of those around you. It's a feeling that everyone can have, but no one can own.

This is what music means to me, and it's a meaning I've tried to share with the little slice of the next generation that I've been lucky enough to be around. I hope they've heard what I threw at them, and I hope they don't take my meaning to be any sort of definition. Minds, bodies, movements, and generations advance by building on what came before. I am hopeful that the little slice I've been around will use the bricks I've thrown at them as a foundation for the future of what music sounds like in the studio, in the living room, and in conversation. They will learn what music means to them.

And that's what music means to me.

Matthew Carron, LICSW

Music, Health, and Well-Being

From a very young age, music has had a profound and visceral effect on me. I remember hearing Bach's "Jesu Joy of Man's Desiring" at five years old. I experienced involuntary tears streaming out of me. My mother, startled, asked what was wrong. I indicated as best I could in the language of a five-year-old that the music was so beautiful it was overwhelming.

We know music impacts the brain in multiple hemispheres, but there is a lot we don't know. What I experience is that every part of my being can sing to a different song, dance to a different beat, and transform with another symphony. If we picture the body like chakras or consider the essential elements of our various human states, primitive, emotional, unconscious dreams, physicality, and spiritual transcendence, music somehow speaks to all of these.

Perhaps music can bring well-being because it occupies all our being?

I am fortunate to play music as a member of Jimmy Buffett's Coral Reefer Band. I wonder at the power of a sound that causes people to fly across the globe to see one of our shows. Something is going on that I don't think we can fully quantify. I make a living sculpting an energy form I don't understand. I am comfortable with that mystery.

Music is something bigger than us. It comes from somewhere inside and outside of us at the same time. At times, it feels as if I am "receiving" the notes when I play music. As if the vibration of everything, including my instrument, gets to speak when we play. With Jimmy Buffett's music, we all end up at the beach together. The band and the audience benefit simultaneously from the shared experience.

In the 1980s, I discovered Brian Eno. His idea that music could be ambient spoke to me. Music has the power to take us somewhere. How can we describe the air of a rainy Spring morning in Paris? Erik Satie "Gymnopédie No. 1" comes to mind. Or the haunting sense of an abandoned train yard in Alton, Illinois, at midnight? The first time I put on Miles Davis' "Kind of Blue," I was there, instantly experiencing immersive loneliness and abandonment, so beautiful I didn't know what to do with it, but I knew I didn't want to leave.

Music heals me and continues to give breath and life to the inexpressible. One of the most beautiful ways to get to know someone when we're dating is to share what music we love and to speak in song. And if I need to grieve the loss of a treasure, music becomes a mysterious light that uncovers what I didn't even know existed within me.

Music connects us. Before the age of 10, my dad, two brothers, and I would sit and listen to music together, not saying a word. Stevie Wonder, Cat Stevens, and many other artists filled the house. Later in our teens, it became a daily ritual to go upstairs to my oldest brother's room and listen to the latest ECM Records Releases. The spatial European Jazz bordered on auditory mysticism. The ECM tagline at that time was something about "The next best thing to silence," which I appreciated for its humility.

What is music? Perhaps the power of its healing is that it speaks to something in us that was there before we had language or even before we were here. It connects to something so much greater than ourselves and yet so personal. It is the healing, the connecting, the experience of knowing and being known, sharing something, anything, including isolation and loneliness.

What I love most about music is that our wholeness starts to return when we become silent and listen.

Jim Mayer
American musician, singer, songwriter,
entrepreneur, children's advocate
Member of Jimmy Buffett's Coral Reefer
Band for over 30 years

Jazz Studies, John Denver, and Clarity

Music is magical, to use an unscientific term. I knew it from an early age. Before I even owned my own radio or cassette player (this was, after all, the 70s), I was learning to play on my grandmother's spinet piano. I was voracious, always eager for more to play, more to learn. When I found a chart on the back page of my beginning piano primer that illustrated the major and minor triads and their variations in every key, I simply memorized it.

But as a listener, I also grew to love the music of that and the preceding generation, just like millions of other people who never played a note did. My hippie-ish uncle began slipping me recordings of Simon & Garfunkel, Crosby, Stills & Nash, James Taylor, Billy Joel, and others, and they became the soundtrack of my gently maturing soul.

Back at the piano, I began to show signs of depth and devotion. I didn't have to be told to practice (well, sometimes). It was more a challenge for teachers to keep up with my appetite than for them to coax me forwards. I performed at Friday morning piano recitals at my elementary school, steamrolling my way into and through Mozart, Beethoven, and eventually Debussy and Copland. I wrote my own piano pieces, simple at first but always experimenting and coopting from the repertoire I'd been exploring.

And on the side, there was my uncle's music, the folk, the singer/songwriter music, the sweet harmonies of the Woodstock era. I found that I could play that too if I put my mind and ear to it. I remembered the triads and other chords from my beginning piano days and began to discover that in them lay the underpinnings of not only the classical music of my studious side but also the 60s and 70s songs that spoke to me in a more personally direct way. I could step away from the serious music of my diligent piano study and, through the music of my "downtime," cultivate something more, well, me.

But piano for me was becoming serious stuff. I was already on to the next thing by my teenage years. A benevolent English teacher had introduced me to jazz, and I was up to my ears in the nuance and technicality of that tradition. I went to college to major in Jazz Studies and spent the next four years (and far beyond) burying myself in upper extension triads, quartal chord voicing, bebop improvisational patterns, and other esoterica. And it all kept me entranced. The innocent music of my childhood, the folksy guitar music and the wide-open spaces of the songs on which I'd grown up faded into background of my life as a driven high-achieving professional musician. I had moved on and left CS&N, JT, and all the rest as a pleasant part of my now-distant musical infancy.

I was tenacious as I made my way into the larger world of performing. Thanks to the demanding and competitive environment I had experienced in college, I now had an arsenal of technical skills at my call. I sat in at local jazz jam sessions and showed off my abilities as an improviser and accompanist. Often under pressure, I honed my sight-reading skills until I had shown myself to be reliable and competent even without any rehearsal. As I developed a positive reputation, I found myself on stage in jazz clubs, tearing through production numbers as a Broadway pit pianist, and even cutting my teeth playing celeste in symphony orchestras. I had become an addict to challenging and usually stressful performance situations. The more mentally exhausting the assignment, the more rewarding the rush. Sixteenth-note syncopations altered dominant harmony, and blisteringly fast tempos had become my drug of choice. I certainly had no space left in my constructed persona for the three-chord "folkie" I had been in my younger incarnation.

Then one day something unexpectedly surfaced to remind from whence I came. I turned on the TV news that morning and was struck by the passage of time – one of the purveyors of the music of my youth had died; the country crooner John Denver was gone in a flying accident. In the post-mortem on the news, "Annie's Song" was playing. Since JD had fallen out of public favor in the 80s, I hadn't heard it in at least fifteen years.

I was transfixed. There is nothing particularly intellectual about the music; it certainly has more to it than some three-chord fare, but it's a simple one-section structure that never leaves the key of D major. But that one section may be the most beautiful 32 bars of music ever composed. The melody is pristine, the lyrics timeless. John's voice on it is clear, honest, exultant.

Hearing that song again after so long, I felt something elusive yet familiar. Maybe the best term for it is "clarity." I had experienced all varieties of positive vibes when playing the music that had become my life-long pursuit. Fulfillment, depth, transcendence, yes, professional accomplishment too, even flat-out goosebumps at times, but this was different. Reliving this relic of my simpler forays into music from back when its magic was first imprinting itself upon me made me feel, to put it simply, just really... good.

I had trained myself to think that the loftier the art, the more rewarding would be my experience. That turns out to not really be the case. I have no regrets about penetrating as deeply into the craft of music as I have in the 50 or so years since I sat on my grandmother's piano bench. But rediscovering the warmth that I felt when first experiencing the magic of music as a young listener has enriched everything I do at the piano. I'm happily honest about where the source of my music lies. It's in there now in everything I play. I guess it always was.

Ben Cook
Associate Professor of Piano, Berklee College of Music
Pianist on hundreds of performances and national
tours with the Boston Pops Orchestra

Music, Songwriting and Community

Baby, baby. I've sung those words before.

Now they mean so much more than just baby, baby.

When you see me baby, will it be a nice surprise?

Will you smile and recognize your Dad's voice, baby?

I wrote that song for Sophie, my first born, within days of knowing Carol was pregnant. Long before I knew she would be a girl or a boy, every day, as often as I could, I would snuggle up next to Carol's pregnant belly and sing. To our first born.

She was already crying when I first held her, within seconds of her being plucked by Caesarian section from her mother's womb. "Sophie, Sophie."

Her eyes opened wide. Her crying stopped. "Sophie. Sophie."

I wrote another song when she first went off to College.

Where I'm going you can't come with me Dad.

I know your sad Dad. I know you're sad.

I'm a-growing and you can't stop me Dad.

Dad, I know you're sad.

But it's my road to travel. To follow or to stray.

Sand. Stone. I'll bear it alone. I may come home.

But not today. Not today.

Music has been a way I have expressed myself since I was seven years old and write my first phrase of music. Cleopatra's tune was in D minor, perhaps reflecting some of what I was going through at the time. And then I was a teenager, falling madly and passionately in love. Every week.

I wrote a lot of songs. Each still can conjure emotions and memories from all those years ago. The excitement of meeting someone for that first time, the hope, the doubt, the first date, the last date, the passion, the sadness, the lesson learnt. Until the next spark.

Each of us probably has some piece of music-memory that activates and transports you back to whatever may have been going on at that moment in your life. And along with that limbic memory are all those limbic emotions, a cataclysm of old feelings welling up *just by hearing a piece of music*. Perhaps even now, reading those last sentences, brought one of those memories to the surface. That's the power of music, right here, and right now.

A song can take me to a sad and dark place, or one of crazy joy! What songs make you feel sad, happy, content? Each one is associated with a time in your life. Each one is a treasure trove of insight. Sometimes I ask my patients if they have a song that means something to them. They may play it on their cellphone, and we use it as a setting for whatever memory they may want to explore.

When I was running an adolescent substance use residential program we had a music room. An old upright piano, a couple of electric keyboards, some percussion. Every now and then we had a patient who played the guitar. The room became a place where all of us could just get away. Some kids would rap, some kids wrote poetry, and another kid would put some music behind it, or another kid would beat-box. We never made a big deal of it, never used it as a springboard for discussion or a group. It was as if we all agreed that this would be a place where people could just express themselves, without having to then figure out the deeper unconscious meaning. It was just to have fun.

Music was brought into groups in other ways. We had some groups with popular music, and we would analyze the lyrics, the kids realizing that perhaps they *had* been influenced by hearing lyrics glorifying using. We looked at some songs of people who had died from using. Every now and then a kid would offer to bring

in some of their own lyrics, which universally were acclaimed and
valued by their peers.

We spent a lot of time exploring music in other ways, especially
in our voices, in the way we talk with each other, or often to each
other or at each other. This music in our language is called prosody:
The patterns of stress and intonation in a language. The word has
its origins in Greek, prosoidia, or song sung to music, tone of a
syllable.

In a group on outsmarting anger, the kids learned that often it
is the *way* you say something that can influence another person,
not just *what* you say. The way those words are said – the tone, the
inflection, the rhythm, can have an enormous influence on whether
the listener feels angry, sad, scared, dismissed, invited, and so many
others. They learned that the way you *feel* about something deeply
influences the way you *say* it, or the way you hear and *interpret*
what is said to you.

Try it yourself. Just say this sentence:

"I am having lasagna for dinner."

Now say the exact same words but as if you like lasagna. Now
if lasagna disgusts you. Amazing isn't it, how the *exact* same words
can have such different meanings, just by the way you say them.

You can inspire jealousy by emphasizing the "I," which could
telegraph that you alone are having lasagna. With the same empha-
sis on the "I," you could also make the person suspicious by imply-
ing that you are trying to take his or her lasagna. The kids in the
group would make the sentence a demand, a question, a joy, a sadness, a plea, a seduction. Amazing, isn't it? The way you say the
words has just as much impact as the words themselves. Human
beings are designed to hear these inflections, the prosody, which
can activate or calm a person's brain.

❋ ❋

When Sophie got married, I chose not to do a father–daughter
dance. I wrote a father–daughter song, which we sang together at
her wedding. It's the little things that matter, it's the little things
you say. That make it fine to go to work and come home every day.
It's the every-day I love you when you wake and fall asleep. It's the
little things that make the day complete.

Now, my youngest child, Becca, is writing music. So much more sophisticated than mine ever was, transporting me back to when I was seven, and tesseracts me far, far into the future. Music is everywhere, a resource that each of us can use, every day, to make our lives complete. For me it is an incredible release to sit at the piano and just play. Perhaps the song I wrote before I even met Sophie. Perhaps the song when I thought Carol and I were breaking up. Perhaps the silly song I wrote called The Eighth Knight of Chanukah. Perhaps a song I wrote long ago but want to play now because I need a way to cry, or to feel elated, or to just relax. Playing the piano and writing music has been a way to connect my inner and outer worlds. It is a melody I hope resonates in anyone who hears it. In my professional life, it is a melody that has helped me to hear and appreciate the music of my patients.

Joseph Shrand, MD

Chief Medical Officer, Riverside Community Care

Founder, Drug Story Theater

Host, Podcast The Dr Joe Show

Poetry and Core Knowledge

In the late 1980s, while walking together down a dirt road in rural Vermont, I asked Robert (Red) Penn Warren, America's first Poet Laureate, "Why poetry?" I wanted to know what it is about poetry that he found so enthralling. He answered that poetry is much like music; when we talk to babies we intuitively break into a "singsong" of rhythmical language and rhyming. Although Red is widely known as the author of *All the King's Men*, he won Pulitzer Prizes in both prose and poetry. He told me he had learned Italian in order to read Dante's *Divine Comedy* in the original tongue, to fully experience the meaning of the poem, as expressed in words, rhythm and rhyme.

As a neurologist I have devoted much of my professional life and personal time studying how the brain serves as the "messenger" of the mind and the world of ideas. I was captivated by Red's response. I recognized that, across cultures, babies appear to be soothed by music, and toddlers' stories are often told in metrical rhymes.

In an attempt to experience the beauty of the untranslated *Commedia*, I studied Italian in my 40s. But I was challenged by having passed the critical period in development, during which the brain effortlessly absorbs a new language; the critical period for language learning closes near puberty, after which it is difficult for most people to acquire a foreign language with a native accent. Nonetheless, for the past thirty-some years I have sought to understand what Red was getting at because I realized he was pointing to something about human nature and, more specifically, how the brain works before cultural experience has modified it. Accordingly, since I could not learn Dante's Italian, I turned to sources that could provide an exegesis of his insights.

Red had suggested that I read TS Eliot, who had a similar great devotion to the language of Dante and recognized the potential of language to convey subtle ideas and meanings. In a book on the impact of Dante on American Letters, Eliot lamented the relative poverty of English as a means for communicating poetically:

> *English is less copiously provided with rhyming words than Italian; and those rhymes we have are in a way more emphatic. The rhyming words call too much attention to themselves: Italian is the one language known to me in which exact rhyme can always achieve its effect – and what the effect of rhyme is, is for the neurologist rather than the poet to investigate.*

But what could a neurologist bring to a discussion of the "exact rhyme can always achieve its effect"?

As I puzzled over this question, one evening I attended a concert of the Boston Symphony Orchestra performing Beethoven's 7th symphony. During the concert, I recognized what happens when we are "pulled along" by the rhythmic rhyming of sound. We mirror the cadence of harmonious sound and are delighted when it becomes faster and louder. We experience a similar pleasure dancing or as we watch a ballet or figure skater perform to music. What joy as I felt my entire body being pulled by the rhythm of the harmony!

As I sat in Symphony Hall, I was reminded of the conversation I had had about poetry with Red and the quotation of Eliot. Babies and toddlers love to be rocked, and to hear the rhythm and rhyming of words. Think of what we do with a child who is crying: we hold, hum or sing, rocking them back and forth, all in rhythmic harmony. The relation of poetry to music became apparent to me. For centuries poetry has been described as "the concrete and artistic expression of the human mind in emotional and rhythmical language." (Encyclopedia Britannica)

Rhythms and pitches found in music in the modern era are recognized to have been present in Sumerian and Babylonian times. A Sumerian love song from over 3,000 years ago is reported to sound like a lullaby, folk song or hymn by a group at UC Berkeley, providing further evidence that meter and scales central to poetry and music are built upon universal principles.

As a neurologist and parent, and through my reading of cognitive scientists who have studied "core knowledge" in infants, we understand that we are not born with our minds a *tabula rasa*, but rather with mental content which exists before post-natal experience has modified the brain. This can be seen in the widespread appeal of lullabies, Mother Goose and Dr Seuss. The aural harmony of both music and poetry likely reflects aspects of our "pre-wired" core knowledge.

So "Why poetry?" As described, poetry has the capacity to engage both emotions and movement but with the addition of language, the intellect can articulate "concrete" ideas. The following excerpt by Encyclopedia Britannica provides an insight into the answer of how the adult mind can be enthralled by poetry:

> When this sea of emotion has "curdled into thoughts," articulate language rhythmically arranged ... can do what no mere wordless music ...[nor] unrhythmical language mortised in a foundation of logic, i.e., prose, can best express ... ideas.

Together, these observations might suggest that great poetry can create synergies, connecting our newly constructed ideas with core knowledge of our brain's pre-experience circuitry. Our experience of great poetry would not be unlike other forms of great Art (painting, architecture, dance, and other art forms), which also can induce a profound sense of awe. This construct may explain the universal appeal of the arts across time and cultures.

Thomas N. Byrne, MD
Professor of Neurology & Health Sciences and Technology
(part-time), Harvard Medical School
Senior Lecturer, Department of Brain and Cognitive Sciences
Massachusetts Institute of Technology

The Power of Music to Connect

I dropped out of medical school to be a musician. Well, at least I tried.

In retrospect, I was not ready to become a doctor, and I avoided class by playing music with a sitarist. He told me about an opening in the Philosophy Department where he was a junior professor. It seemed like a great opportunity, even though I only took two philosophy courses in college.

My Dean refused to let me withdraw, told me to take my time, study anything remotely relevant to medicine, and put me in an MD, PhD program. Reluctantly, I agreed. It turned out to be the best decision I ever made. And I'm forever grateful to him.

Academia was dreadfully sterile. After two years, I re-entered medical school. But those two years gave me the chance to hang out and play with other musicians – not for money, but for fun. Those hours and hours of just making music changed my life. I learned to listen. I learned to play what came to me in the moment. I learned not to be scared to play the wrong note. And most of all, I learned how to connect with others and make them sound good.

Fast forward about 15 years. I became a doctor and had 4 kids. Now 8 grandkids.

What's most precious to me and my family is sitting in a living room around the piano singing with a bunch of friends. It's a holiday tradition. There would be no Thanksgiving or any other celebration without our getting out the guitars and any other available instruments.

Mind you, it's not always pretty. Our harmonies are usually off. Our timing is generally poor. But we get wrapped up in it and go on most of the night. Everyone feels great – and we're feeling it together. That's the magic of music.

Gene Beresin, MD, MA
Executive Director, The Clay Center for Young Healthy Mind at
The Massachusetts General Hospital
Professor of Psychiatry, Harvard Medical School
Band member, Pink Freud and The Transitional Objects

Music Is Magic

We used to "shun-pike" when we were small. That would entail getting 6 members of our family into a wood paneled station wagon to ride along the old country roads going nowhere other than to take in the natural beauty of the countryside with all its harvested crops and animals. It wasn't just a ride though. Inside the vehicle, there was a symphony of voices with the driver, my father, the conductor. His hands were simultaneously in the air to lead the songs and on the steering wheel to make sure we were going in the right direction.

The tunes were not "Old McDonald Had a Farm," but were the songs of the 30s and 40s such as *Heart of My Heart, Moonlight Bay, Bill Bailey, The Dark Town Stutter's Ball* and many more. Each family member knew every word to every song and belted those songs out as if we were participating in a Broadway Show. Music became part of our DNA.

I remember one Christmas morning when I entered our living room there were a plethora of gifts scattered around the room. To the right, there was also a beautiful new piano with a large red bow waiting to be played. I was elated even though the piano came with many expectations and subsequent, tedious piano lessons in the years that followed. It was the beginning of my formal musical training.

There were many memorable house parties that our parents hosted. My father (the conductor) would shout out to me (regardless of what I was involved in) to come into the party, sit down on the piano bench and play the "keys" while he sang with abandon with or without the guests. He was a combination of Frank Sinatra and Louie Armstrong. Those were the days as music was at the core of festive family gatherings.

Fast forward to chorus in High School then off to camp in the summertime... fêted with non-stop music, singing, dancing, learning to play the guitar, camp musicals and more. My repertoire grew exponentially.

Then off to college to study education and to use my musical aptitude to connect with elementary age children in Colorado. It was the 70s. Music defined our culture with Woodstock, John Denver – Rocky Mountain High, James and Livingston Taylor, Bonnie Raitt and so many others. I remember sitting down at a piano in a classroom where I was student teaching. All the K-1 students in our class gathered around and began singing every song I played. It felt magical, powerful, and developed a true sense of wonder for me as I was communicating with students in a new and more effective way than anything I had ever learned or tried before.

Throughout my 30-year career in education, I used music to communicate with children of all ages. I used songs, chants and poems to teach different subjects in the K-4th grade classes. There were songs to promote community building, songs to address peace in the world, and songs to help learn grammar, geography, and math. Music would provide safe and organized transitions in the early childhood programs and playgroups that I led for parents and toddlers. Many of the participants in our playgroups were non-English speaking and the songs were instrumental in helping them to acquire new and stronger language skills. Music, rhythm and repetition invigorated, uplifted, enlightened, relaxed, calmed, empowered, focused and soothed the souls of each student and that of their parents.

For students who had learning challenges, to the children with higher level academic abilities, music created an equal playing field for all. It was a way to foster creativity, introspection and connectedness. I wrote musicals using age-appropriate literature, familiar music with rewritten lyrics to accompany the themes of the stories, a venue that made acting, speaking and singing accessible to all and a feeling of success that each participant could experience.

From 1987 to 1992, my youngest brother was on a journey living with HIV/AIDS. During his final year, when hospitalized for cancer treatment, he would be ushered off for various tests and with a twinkle in his eye he would look back at us and say... please sing my song! "His song" became the theme song for my entire family's journey with HIV/AIDS. The song was *This Little Light of Mine*. I'd have my guitar by his hospital bed each time he had to stay there and regardless of who was in the room, we (family and friends) would sing. My brother loved the music and through his fear, the pain and the uncertainty about his future, music helped to heal and provide strength and comfort.

After my brother's death, a foundation was started to educate others about HIV/AIDS.

Through the foundation, an ecumenical Seder of Hope and Healing began and lasted for 15 years. It was held at our local synagogue for people all over Boston affected by HIV/AIDS. My brother's "song" would be sung at the end of the evening with 400+ people holding handles in a circle. Each person was filled with hope, and many were living with the disease as they passed a lit candle hand to hand around the room and sang *This Little Light of Mine*.

Music is the universal language that connects us all. It helps us to slow us down when we are feeling energetic or frantic. It helps to uplift us when we are feeling melancholy or blue and it adds joy to our lives when needed.

Music is in my heart and soul. When I use my guitar or ukulele to sing with children who come into my life from time to time, I see in their eyes a form of communication and joy that I can't access in any other way. They say that a person's eyes are the window into their soul. I feel that through the music I share with others, the soul becomes more transparent and the connection with one another becomes deeper and more meaningful.

Music is indeed magical.

Debbie Felllman

Advisory Board Member, the MGH Clay Center

Former Elementary School Teacher (K-4),

Music/Literacy Instructor, and Co-Director, Parent-

Child Home Program, Brookline Public Schools.

BRIEF INTRODUCTION

This vignette was written by my 13-year-old grandson, Zeke. As you can see from his contribution, his beautiful writing, introspection and understanding of how music affects his well-being are quite

extraordinary for his age. I say this objectively and not simply because
I am his grandfather (though I am biased)! I have no doubt, he will
become an incredible music producer, should he choose this as a career.

My Own Therapy Session

Before I talk about music, let's talk about me. While that might
come off as narcissistic to some, music and its effects on your mental health are so singular and personal that *not* giving you a brief
look into my life would be like only showing you half of the picture. Even before I had the ability to decide what music I liked,
my parents would frequently play their favorite albums or songs,
whether it would be on speakers in the house or blasting through
the stereo in our white Volvo. And it wasn't for me specifically but
rather for their own enjoyment and pleasure. They weren't trying
to show me or teach me anything, but ended up doing so anyway,
as I was given an opportunity to listen and experience a wide variety of genres and styles for myself. As I grew a bit older and began
picking music for myself, I would put into the CD player whatever
I enjoyed at the time and sit in front of it for an hour or longer,
slowly watching the song number tick up and let the music flow
through me. It was almost a form of meditation, a way to relax and
enjoy myself. I didn't know it back then, but I was already using
music as a source of relaxation and simple pleasure.

For a while, that's all I got out of music. My sister and I would
beg our father to put on a playlist of songs we'd set up, and if he
complied, we'd sit there, listening and singing along to pop stars
like Katy Perry and Taylor Swift. Music, to me, was just something
that made you smile. And for the time being, that was perfectly
fine. When my family moved away from proximity to my school
but didn't want to switch to a new one, the long drive into the city
was made tolerable by our mom. She would give my sister and me
the aux and allow us to play whatever we wanted, no matter how
many times we repeated a song or played Selena Gomez over and
over again. Music had evolved into a technique or preparation for
school, a little dose of enjoyment before inevitable boredom.

Around March 2020, as I assume you know, the world shut
down. Remote school made my mental state slowly start to sink,

and I started to resort to - you guessed it - music, as a therapy of sorts. As I look back on my favorite artists of the time, I realize they were all very dark, depressing, and inward-looking. Music had turned into my consolation, my way of telling myself that other people felt the same things I did.

I was young then, and I still am. I'm at a stage of my life where my musical taste is expanding rapidly, and that's exactly what happened over the last two years. As I started feeling better after my depression during lockdown, I started listening to more things, developing a love for genres like hip-hop and soul and rock. I started getting into producing, making my own beats inspired by the artists and songs I liked so much. I started experimenting with Garage Band.

Now, I'm making my own beats in Logic, and listening to artists like MF DOOM, J Dilla, Kendrick Lamar, Radiohead, and Earl Sweatshirt on a daily basis. I'm only 13, and what music does for my well-being is sure to change. But at the present day, I use music as a guide. It's music I go to when I feel down, music I make and feel a sense of pride, music I love discussing and talking about. It's music that really keeps me going throughout the day and wake up tomorrow with a smile on my face. Music helps me get through my life, and I hope it will continue being able to do that.

Zeke Braman
Avid music fan, budding producer and rapper

Through the Doorways of Music

Music happens for me in a combination of place, people, and meaning.

One of my early memories is standing in my parent's living room by a heavy piece of furniture that made music. It was a Sylvania Walnut AM/FM Stereo Record Player. To a kid, the thing approximated about half the size of my dad's car. I was in.

And boy, could it make music.

I played Santana's first album *Abraxas* hundreds of times. *Oy Como Va. Black Magic Woman.*

I got a hold of the record when a kid in my 5th grade class asked what I wanted for my birthday. "A record," I said. Which sounded reasonable, until he came back a few days later. "My mother wants to know which record you want." I remembered Santana on the radio going to school, and said, "A record by Santana."

The polyrhythms flowing from that gigantic piece of furniture would transform me. Over and over and over – the guitar playing, the whistle blowing, the percussion – all of it opened doors that never would never close.

How Carlos' music got to a young kid growing up in the hills of Louisville, Kentucky is the story of music. Carlos was born in Autlán de Navarro, Jalisco, Mexico. He played violin first at 5, and then guitar at 8.

His compositions as a 21-year-old filled a yellow Kentucky public school bus that would then migrate onto that Sylvania Walnut Stereo Record Player. For me, the sounds of Santana in my family's living room was my youth. It reminds me of friends and football games and BB guns. Of the beautiful brown-haired girl Susan McElwaine who wore jeans and lived up the hill. It took me out of my culture into a land of strange sounds that integrated all of the restless energies that made no sense. "Oy Como Va" is "How's it going?" in Spanish. "Always good" was the answer when that circle of wax was on. I considered Santana home – and his percussion guitar sounds – the beginning of music and connection that mattered.

Similar to seeing the cover of The Beatles *Rubber Soul* and those distorted mop-top faces on a free summer day for the first time. *I've Just Seen a Face*, *In My Life*, and *Norwegian Wood* brought their British, boyish rock sensibility to a southern youthful knoll, and helped me and my friends become what we were. No one had written like that or sung like that. Growing up was clearly about something much bigger than the gears on my bicycle and our basketball court in the driveway. There was a lot going in the world, and those songs would transport me through the voices of handsome young Brits to visions that were far beyond the woods by our house.

> *There are places I'll remember. All my life though some have changed. Some forever not for better. Some have gone and some remain. All these places had their moments. With lovers and friends, I still can recall. Some are dead and some are living. All my life, I've loved them all.*

Who wrote like that? What must it be like to be a 27-year-old John? Something about the sunshine on the record on that knoll created a calling – a doorway.

I was sitting in my business school dorm room decades later, imagining a music store where musicians would tell their stories of the music, the shelves would tell the stories of Louis Armstrong, and the many innovators who got us there. People would come to hear them talk about the power of the creative process. "If you build it."

We opened the first Hear Music store in Berkeley California November 1992. The greats came to inaugurate a new kind of music experience. Dave Grisman, Mark O'Connor, Jonathan Richmond and other acoustic legends played a free concert for thousands who assembled and poured through the store. We closed 4th Street, and opened the store on a vision of a new kind of music experience. Music stores would never be the same.

Inside, Ry Cooder, Joni Mitchell, Bonnie Raitt, Ray Charles – alongside dozens of other musical visionaries–guided you to sounds that inspired them. The experience built on their words, their voices, their sounds. We projected artists' quotes on integrated-plaster walls. *Elle Magazine* called it like "dying and going to music heaven." *National Public Radio* wondered how the experience had not existed before. We set the music landscape on fire with a new sensibility of discovery – an audience discovering place, people, and meaning behind the transformative musicians, compositions, and artists. The VH1 senior team told me later that much of what we did at Hear Music informed the network's approaches and essential culture. Place and people and connection began to congeal to set music in its fullness – in its true landscape – where it comes from, and where it is going.

The store was a transformative waterfall of desire, harmony, stories, grace, musicians, healers, survivors, adventurers, and people. And people would come from all over the Bay Area to help make the transcendence.

I remember standing in the store, and 2 women marveled as John Lee Hooker sang *The Healer* from his recent release, with a quote from John Lee about the song appearing on the integrated-plaster wall. I explained to them how we did it – a Kodachrome slide projector synced to the latest digital CD changer–song by song by song.

I smile now remembering that Carlos Santana played guitar with John Lee Hooker on the track. From that walnut cabinet in Louisville, Kentucky to the in-store play in Berkley, California, the legacy of music's healing power came to produce Hear Music's compilations by The Rolling Stones, Ry Cooder, KD Lang, Tony Bennett, Joni Mitchell, Yo Yo Ma, Ray Charles, and many more, on our *Artist Choice* series where artists led you to great artists. Artist Choice found a geography and language in which we could share music's healing power in many forms from many cultures.

The process is about finding a place in your imagination large enough to capture it all.

J. Kevin Sheehan,
Founder of Hear Music
Co-Founder Hope Collaborative
Co-Founder LeaderJam LLC

Music in Treatment

As a musician in long-term recovery, I played music for many years searching for ways to describe how I felt in the inside. I recall finding my calling at the age of 7 when I took piano lessons. My mother was a classically trained vocalist. I enjoyed all forms of music from musicals, opera, and by the age of 10, I fell head over heels for The Beatles.

It wasn't long after that I started using substances. I found my first real high at the age of 14 when I discovered wine at my friend's bar mitzvah. This was around the time that I discovered Bob Dylan, David Bowie, and this new guy from Boston named James Taylor.

I quickly graduated from alcohol to cannabis.

I gravitated toward other stimulants and narcotics in high school. My own experience with substance use became more significant as I dealt with losing my brother to substance use, mental health, and suicide when I was 16. It was in October around the time of my birthday. I didn't see it coming but wasn't surprised. I think we were both asking for help, but no one picked up on our cry for help.

Music became my language and means to survive, make a living, to feed the need to express my feelings. I am not sure how I passed school. It was such a blur.

Music became a priority for my existence until my substance use took over. I left my hometown with a plan to follow my passion and play music. I somehow ended up in Boston and then Los Angeles in the early 80s signed to a recording contract. I continued to mix my experience with alcohol, cannabis, and narcotics to cope with the deeper covert issues of sadness and loss. The important thing was that I was playing music.

It was a sad day when I faced the reality that I was playing music for the purpose of feeding my addictions. I was very discouraged to face the fact that I was not as good as I knew I could be and had compromised my creative self, drowning in feelings of hopelessness, caught up in the perception that substances were helping me be a better artist.

I wasn't my best.

Years into my recovery, I continue to use music and songwriting to express how I feel as a person in recovery that music was, is, and will always be my language. Music was the priority on my journey to the debts of my addiction. It is now the voice of recovery. My way of expressing my heart and soul.

I opened the doors of Right Turn with the help of Dr Anne Alonso in March of 2003. My goal was to incorporate evidence-based treatment along with complementary therapies of music and art for the treatment of substance use disorder and dual diagnosis issues.

We found that experiential therapies of music and art served as a tool of engagement which allowed individuals and their families identify with the need to access the wounded child and desire to recover the loss of a creative side which was hijacked by substance use. I also want to recognize that the use of music and art therapy is a process for individuals to develop a language to talk about deeper covert issues and trauma. I have found that often individuals have traumatic experiences that are preverbal, rendering them hopeless, and without language or verbal skills to speak about what they are experiencing.

Music services as a delivery system to identify and communicate hidden feelings that some people just don't want to talk about. It is likely they don't have the vocabulary to speak and define their experience. People tend to self-medicate these feelings for long periods of substance use and need to find a safe place to begin the process of talking about covert depression and trauma. Music is a language that they use.

Woody Giessmann, LADC-I, CADC, CIP, AIS
Founder of Right Turn and Addiction Specialist
Professional Musician, former drummer for the Del Fuegos

Music as Healing

When I was a little girl, we never ate dinner in the dining room. That was because we had a Steinway baby grand piano in there which took up most of the room! It wasn't played much but it was just a part of the room. Every once in a while, my Dad would have his musical friends over to play Big Band music and I remember those evenings fondly. My Dad played the sax, and the clarinet and Russ Mock played the piano. My Dad left us when I was 12 and took the piano with him.

My mother loved piano concertos, especially the big ones, and I grew up listening to them on the stereo in the living room. I took violin in 4th grade and loved it but gave it up when it was no longer "cool" to play an instrument. When I met my husband at age 15, he played guitar and sang folk music. This was in the 60s of course. He had a beautiful voice! It was part of why I fell in love with him.

Over the years I have continued to listen to and love music of all kinds. When pregnant with my son I was obsessed with Mozart piano concertos and listened to them constantly. My husband and I would listen to WCRB classical music station every morning while getting ready for work.

It turned out that my son became a professional musician, just now finishing up a master's degree in Music Therapy. So, I have been surrounded by music my whole life but never really played anything beyond the violin for a couple of years when I was young. I always felt that a house was not a home unless it had a piano in it. About 20 years ago my husband bought us a beautiful Yamaha Clavinova piano which fits easily into our tiny house.

For years no one played it! My son, while musical, was playing drums, guitar and trombone. At some point he started playing the piano on his own and I was thrilled to have it used. I would look at it and say, "I wish I could play the piano!" But I was afraid that I would fail and not be able to learn. I also imagined playing beautiful classical music and had no interest in beginner pieces. So, I looked longingly at my lovely piano without touching it.

Three years ago, my husband was diagnosed with leukemia. It was a difficult and stressful time. About two years ago I was looking at the piano and said to myself,

"I don't want to be on my deathbed and be thinking that I wished I had learned to play the piano!" I decided right then that I would find a teacher. My son knew the perfect person, a lovely young man who is a composer, music therapist and piano teacher.

I have been taking lessons once every two weeks for the past two years. It has changed my life in so many ways! I found that I worked through the beginner books very quickly and it gave me a new sense of accomplishment I didn't expect. I play every day if even for a few minutes but sometimes for hours. Within months I was able to play what I refer to as "real music" – simple Chopin and Bach. I especially love Robert Schumann's Album for the Young.

What I have found is that because it is so hard to learn to read music and play the piano, when I am practicing, I can't focus on anything else. This means that other worries and problems recede, and I go completely into the music. It is challenging and rewarding and soothing and relaxing all at the same time. It reduces stress and I believe that stress causes disease. I cannot imagine my life without a piano anymore.

My husband, sadly, died six months ago. It has been a very difficult time for me. He suffered greatly before his death, and I have been dealing with the loss of a 55-year relationship as well as the trauma of watching him suffer. I find that at times my focus is not as good when I sit down to play but I have continued with my lessons and my playing, and it is healing. When I am lonely or stressed, I play, and it helps. I am never really alone as long as I have my music. I am drawn to minor keys and find that they mirror my mood. Rather than make me feel worse, it often feels better to let the mood run free. I truly feel that music is therapy for me, and I am so very grateful to have realized this and acted upon it. I am grateful to my husband and my son and my teacher for encouraging me and believing I could do it. It brings great joy and healing into my life every day.

Sandy Peck, Ed.M. RD
Educator and
Life-long Learner

Cancer and Music for Resilience

Cancer is a funny disease. You don't necessarily feel ill, but a routine yearly test can go south and you are on the ride of your life, perhaps for your life. In my case, I was 49 years old.

Cancer has its own world in the hospital. It tends to have the newest interior design, banks of supportive social workers, nurses, volunteers, therapists and doctors, softer colors, more upholstered furniture. Going through those doors made me feel like I did when I bridged as a Brownie to become a Girl Scout. I was now entering a different world. In this world, my husband and daughter (thankfully) didn't live. It was one that I didn't want to be a part of but one that was empathic, hopeful, desperate, winning, losing and very, very real.

The Surgery Experience

After several surgeries during the summer, my husband and I were scheduled to go to Switzerland for my 50th birthday. I had been saving money for this trip for years and the surgeries had now put it into doubt. Would I be able to fly? Would I be able to hike? I spent the summer trying to put myself in the best possible position for these surgeries so that I could have a strong recovery.

To achieve that aspiration, I dedicated myself to practicing the Relaxation Response (RR). The RR describes when your body is functioning in a state of rest and restoration rather than in the opposite state of fight-or-flight, also known as the stress response. To achieve this response, one follows a practice that triggers your brain to release chemicals and signals that slow down your metabolism. This practice is an intentional engagement with the inner peace circuitry of your brain.

I created a playlist of music that I titled "surgery- relaxation." I told the anesthesiologist that I would be practicing the RR and to minimize the anesthesia. Since the research was done at the prestigious Mass General, anesthesiologists were aware of it. I just wish they would promote it more and routinize it.

The music worked like a charm. I was very relaxed and did well with the first two surgeries. For the third, I was struggling mightily. I was to have a disfiguring surgery and was crying in the pre-op area. Having waited all day for a 1 pm surgery time was very difficult and the tears I held inside were spilling over. The anesthesiologist, who apparently doesn't tolerate crying, plunged the catheter syringe saying 'here comes the happy juice.' I woke hours later after the surgery disoriented, confused and without the ability to remember what was said to me. The amnesia would persist for several days. It was scary.

I definitely prefer music and the right amount of anesthesia to do the job. That was too much.

Because of a wonderful surgery experience and a good recovery, my husband and I took off for our wonderful, much anticipated hiking trip in Switzerland. I felt triumphant and heartened that I had come through this cancer scare so well. I attributed much of it to my practice of the Relaxation Response with music.

Chemotherapy

When we returned, I was to see the oncologist that I had met at the beginning of the diagnostic process. During that initial visit, she said I would need to have chemotherapy. The surgeon however had said she "got it all" and that I would not need chemo. New research put me in the grey area of choice here. I was heartened by this news. But the oncologist, one of Boston's finest, would have nothing to do with that. She was adamant that I would need chemotherapy and pointed her finger at me saying

I can get you through this. And if you don't take this treatment now, you will come back in 5 years and be metastatic and I won't have anything for you.

It was devastating news. The chemotherapy would last for 15 months.

Enter my life in an infusion suite. Chemotherapy is what binds all of the various cancers together- colon, lung, prostate, etc. We all come together to sit for infusions that can last up to 8 hours. How will you spend that time? All that was available to us for entertainment and engagement were televisions. Why would anybody want to watch programs like Jerry Springer during chemotherapy? Lots of folks did but that was not what I wanted to do.

As much as I dreaded the drugs, I thought how wonderful it would be to have "time off." I also felt that I needed to fill that gift of time with esthetic beauty and laughter. At the time, I had been teaching and working many various contracts. And I would have to keep working through my treatments because my husband and I were paying for our healthcare benefits out of pocket. There was no time off, no disability insurance for backup. I would make these hours a gift to myself.

I gathered together my chemo resources – a guitar or ukulele, DVDs of operas, comedies and the 1985/1986 world series of the Boston Celtics (a wildly happy blast from the past). I brought along art supplies and spent time making art to different pieces of music. My bedside table was an altar and my dear husband brought me favorite foods for lunch (no grilled cheese on white bread served on and under plastic). I had a computer to access YouTube videos of favorites as well as the Web. I watched lots of films of Ella Fitzgerald, Renee Fleming, Louis Armstrong, Johnny Carson and David Byrne. I asked and almost all of the time was infused in a private room (there were only two). There I could make music and laugh out loud, not feeling that I had to stifle it in anyway. I actually looked forward to those days of indulging rest and restoration.

My First Day

Once in a restaurant a waiter asked me if I was having chemo. I was grey and wearing a turban. I certainly couldn't hide it. When I said, "yes" he said that his mother was having chemo and called it her "rat poison." I couldn't think of it like that even if that is what the chemicals are. If the chemo was going to do its best work, I wanted to be in the Relaxation Response and to pepper that with lots of laughter. I wanted my external as well as my internal environments to be clean, tended, supported, and nourished. I wanted to maximize the effect the drugs had and not impede them by being stressed and negative.

I remember these days warmly, as being some of the sweetest days I have had. They were swaths of time to practice self-care deeply and I had so little of that in my busy life. And these days were filled, truly filled with the beauty and power of music in ways that were undeniable. I listened to music prescriptively throughout this long experience and can't imagine getting through it without this powerful resource for resilience.

It wasn't all upbeat. There were times that I was so very sick. There were times that I became discouraged and didn't feel like I wanted to continue. So, I created a touchstone song, a special song that I could sing when I sorely needed courage. That song was *You'll never walk alone*. On the morning of a treatment day when I felt despaired, I would let myself be as unhappy as I needed to, alone in my bedroom. I would then emerge, singing this beloved song both internally or externally. I would then get in the car and go and do what I had to do. The song was a constant reminder that I was not alone, that friends and family were with me. In addition, I could picture all the researchers that developed the drugs, the carriers that delivered the drugs to the hospital's pharmacy, the pharmacists that filled it and the volunteer that transported it to the oncology department. I didn't know them, but I always blessed them.

In the words of Plato, music brought "wings to the mind, flight to the imagination, and charm and gaiety to life and to everything." I was encouraged and emboldened, I was vulnerable and comforted. Such is the power and beauty of music.

In my last chemo session, my beloved friends and music therapy colleagues came to "sing me home." The room was filled with music – we could hardly get the IV poles in the room. I was overwhelmed with their love and the joy they created. It was more then I felt I deserved which had me on my knees in gratitude. Here we are blessings the meds and those who created it and administer it.

Ten years later, my oncologist likes to say I'm cured. Having been through it once, I know there is no free pass here. I have joined a new tribe, a good and noble tribe and there is no going back. When I look upon those days, I remember them fondly. I felt loved and cared for. I felt courageous and despaired, alone and supported, calm and anxious. In addition to the loving care that my husband and friends provided, I had the beauty and power of music to fill my days and to fill my heart.

What is your song list for vulnerable times? What makes you feel calm when you are anxious? What makes you feel brave when you are frightened? What makes you feel hopeful when you are despaired? What songs will accompany your joys and your sorrows? The possibilities are endless.

Kathleen M Howland. PhD
Music Therapy (MT-BC. NMT/F)
Speech Therapy (CCC-SLP)
LSVT Certified
Faculty, Berklee College of Music

The Power of a Guitar

"Illness is the night side of life, a more onerous citizenship. Everyone who is born holds dual citizenship, in the kingdom of the well and in the kingdom of the sick. Although we all prefer to use the good passport, sooner or later each of us is obliged, at least for a spell, to identify ourselves as citizens of that other place."

~ *Susan Sontag*

In 2001, I was the mom of a teenage son who played a mean guitar, could hold his own on a drum set, fronted a band with his friends, and soloed in the jazz band at school, Nick had also just been diagnosed with cancer of the bile ducts, a rare and usually fatal disease. A life that was overflowing with friends, music, and unlimited possibility rapidly disappeared as hospital stays, radiation therapy, chemotherapy, surgeries and scans soon enveloped Nick and our family. Nick's world as a musician, a lacrosse player, a student leader came to a screeching halt as what was most important to him and gave him joy vanished.

Music was central to Nick from an early age. A precocious child, he was fascinated by the Beatles much to the chagrin of preschool and kindergarten teachers who tried to steer him toward more traditional kid singers and songs, like *Wheels on the Bus* when he was much more interested in *Yellow Submarine*. By the time he was in first grade, Nick was recording mix tapes of Beatles songs for family members with his own running commentary on the songs and lyrics. In retrospect, his study of the Beatles and their music introduced him to an ambiguous, complex and challenging world well beyond his years. Nick got his first electronic drum set while in preschool, but soon envisioned himself as much more John Lennon than Ringo Starr. Nick learned all he could about playing the guitar, forming bands with friends and performing with panache on the stage with the middle school jazz band.

As parents, when your child is diagnosed with a life-limiting illness you quickly move into survival mode. Your world becomes focused on finding a way for your child to survive their illness. Survival is key to everything you think about night and day. My husband and I immersed ourselves in researching and obtaining the most state of the art medical and surgical treatment protocols and interventions and assembled a dream team of highly acclaimed medical specialists at one of the nation's premier academic medical centers. Nick's cancer treatment consisted of multiple inpatient stays, and when able to go home, returning to the hospital for twice a day outpatient radiation therapy, chemotherapy and frequent blood transfusions. Nick had a catheter placed in his chest to provide nutrition and medication. Nick suffered severe side effects of both his disease and its treatment. With his immune system compromised, protecting him from normal environmental germs became paramount. Several weeks into his treatment Nick said to my husband Paul and me "I just want to be a kid again." In that moment we recognized that we had all become unintended citizens of the kingdom of the sick without a map or a way to navigate back to the kingdom of the well, even for a short visit. It then became so obvious what needed to happen – Nick needed to be part of his world again, he needed his guitars, and he needed to make music.

One memorable night, after Nick had been readmitted to the hospital, I walked into his room to find his doctor, an esteemed senior leader in the field of pediatrics, with feet propped up on Nick's bed, simply listening to a 14-year-old riff some Beatles tune on his prized turquoise hollow bodied electric guitar – it was magical. For me, it was a lasting gift of the recognition of the healing power of music for all of us in the room that night. The simple, yet profound act of making and listening to music connected us all in a universal experience – and for that bit of time Nick received his passport back to the kingdom of the well. Nick died a few weeks later, but the incredible healing that music brought him and those around him remain indelible in our minds. Beatles music still plays in our house. connecting us to a boy gone much too soon and reminding us that a guitar can be powerful medicine.

Pamela Katz Ressler, MS. RN, HNB-BC
Founder Stress Resources, Concord Massachusetts
Assistant Clinical Professor Tufts University School of Medicine
in Public Health and Community Medicine

A Hospital Musician from Nashville

A music group in the 1960s called "The Lovin' Spoonful" wrote a song extolling the many virtues of musicians from Nashville, especially guitar players. It was called *Nashville Cats*. As a teen, aspiring guitarist, I loved the song. Decades later, as a hospice and palliative care doctor in an academic hospital in Portland, Oregon, I met a patient who was a guitarist from Nashville, and my love and appreciation for that song increased many-fold.

Patients are musicians too, playing or listening. They've picked a guitar once or twice, and music might touch them. It might treat their symptoms and move beyond that to helping to understand the present, true hope, and the threat of death.

As a palliative care doctor, I spent a lot of time on the cancer wards, 13K and 14K. Occasionally, walking into a patient's room, I would notice a guitar. This would be the kind of thing that might cause a rounding "team" of oncologists, surgeons, etc. to comment "Oh you brought your guitar! Must feel a lot more like home. Now let me tell you about your latest scan." That is, if the team even noticed the guitar – which was not a sure thing.

But the guitar by the bed always seemed to me like what Dr Parker J. Palmer would call a "third thing." A third thing carries a potential invitation into a deeper conversation by means of a nonthreatening, but meaningful item or concept that both patient and doctor can easily talk about. I would ask open-ended questions about the guitar, what kind of music the patient liked to play, how long they had been playing, whether they wrote music, and so on. Then I would politely ask if I could pick up the guitar. The answer was always yes, usually an enthusiastic yes.

If the answer was less than enthusiastic I would just pick up the guitar, look at it, compliment it, and put it back in case.

If the answer was enthusiastic, I would make sure that the guitar was in tune, play a D major chord, add a couple of notes, and try to make the tone as beautiful as I could. The Russian composer, Scriabin, thought that the D chord was yellow. While I don't share his synesthesia, and I don't think I'm as crazy as people thought he was, I agree that the D chord sounds yellow to me – a beautiful sonic color for a room on a cancer ward.

After a few minutes of music and conversation about music and guitars, our conversation turned to deeper thoughts, hopes, fears, and dreams about life-limiting illness, family, and suffering in all its forms.

Once, it did not end there.

A patient with what turned out to be incurable cancer had moved from Nashville, Tennessee with his ancient dog and his partner to be near his two daughters. His partner was in the room along with these daughters, and they were a beautiful, blended, supportive family. His lovely guitar was there, too. The patient had worked for the forestry service, spending much of his work life in a canoe, going up and down the rivers of Tennessee, checking on the health of the forests.

He was an excellent guitarist, a darn good singer, and he had musical charisma. He was a warm and friendly extrovert who had developed his own set of musical friends in Portland Oregon over just a few months.

He invited me to come to a song circle at his house.

I went.

There were seven of us in the circle. The patient's dog had the most severe case of arthritis I had ever seen in any animal, human or non-human. The dog could barely walk, but like most dogs, he gave no sign of self-pity or complaint. He just limped around, dragging a leg, looking up at us, paying careful attention, and thereby becoming a part of the circle and a part of the music.

We went around the circle about five times, each of us having to choose a song that we would lead, while the others followed along.

There's no way to really talk about the power of this gathering without reciting maudlin, over-used, meaningless clichés. But perhaps the simplest way to express the feeling produced by the music and love inside and outside that circle is to say that it was transcendent.

This wonderful musical, dying man was something like the human analog of his sweet dog... uncomplaining, attentive, with a dog/Buddha nature.

He was a patient on the hospice that I directed. He died. The music did not.

++++++++++++++++++++++++++++++++++++++

But it's not all good. On the 13th floor of the hospital where I worked, (13K) housed the solid tumor patients, where I met the man from Tennessee.

Two days a week there's a woman who comes with a big hammer dulcimer. She sets it up in the hallway, where it can potentially be heard in all 30 of the rooms.

I am constitutionally unable to tune music out. I must listen carefully. More than once, I would be walking down the hall, talking to somebody, and the hammer dulcimer would start playing a hammer dulcimer version of Led Zeppelin's "Stairway to Heaven."

> *"Listen," I would say." Do you hear that song?" Usually the person I was with would not have noticed it. I was hoping that the patients would not be singing along to themselves. The only stairway from 13th floor (to heaven) would lead to the 14th floor, which is the leukemia and bone marrow transplant unit– where patients are even sicker than they are on the 13th floor. And closer to heaven.*

> *This was just plain weird. I spoke to a couple of people, but I just didn't have the heart to speak to this musical volunteer, to recommend that she avoid playing "Stairway to Heaven."*

It's obviously a challenging song on the hammer dulcimer, and I'm sure that she worked hard to learn it.

The only music I ever heard that was more disturbing, was when I worked at Beth Israel Hospital in New York City. There was a 14-bed inpatient palliative care unit there, and one day a string quartet from Juilliard came to play for the patients. They played an adaptation of Ravel's" Pavane for a Dead Princess." I found myself hoping that no patient or family member on the floor knew this music.

Music is my path to peace. It has the potential for beauty and abstraction in a world cluttered with abstractions masquerading as facts: serum osmolality, or anion gap, for example.

In my high school yearbook I chose a quote from the Indian poet Tagore, "music fills the infinite between two souls." It's embarrassingly adolescent. But it's also sort of true.

If there is any way to introduce beauty into the lives, and the consciousness of anyone, especially those facing life-limiting illness, or death, that is where I want to be. That is where doctors ought to be. Doctors, nurses, social workers, respiratory therapists, those who sweep and dust and mop, all of us: let's all see if we can bring a flash of yellow, real yellow, into these grey-brown-black rooms. Remember, our dogs are there already.

Eric Walsh, MD
Emeritus Professor of Family Medicine
Oregon Health Sciences University

Billy

Billy was 28 years old when I met him in 1989. I was asked to see him to seek any possible neurological explanation for the chronic catatonic state in which he had remained for the previous eight years. He had been examined by some of the most prominent psychiatrists in the region, had had trials of antidepressants, neuroleptics and mood stabilizers, and had had trials of electroconvulsive therapy (ECT) three times. Although he began to move more normally for about two weeks following two of these ECT series, he soon reverted to a nearly motionless state, requiring hand-over-hand feeding and eventual placement in a group home. Four years after symptom onset an electroencephalogram (EEG) revealed a pattern mildly suggestive of partial seizures. His residential staff reported two episodes of staring and incontinence. Trials of four different anticonvulsants at therapeutic levels produced no improvement.

Billy had Down syndrome and was moderately intellectually disabled. Prior to his illness he'd enjoyed competing in Special Olympics and going horseback riding. There was a history of bipolar mood disorder in a cousin and severe Obsessive Compulsive Disorder (OCD) in a sibling. His family clearly dated the onset of his illness to the days following an accident that had occurred when he was 17. He had been fooling around in the kitchen and accidentally bumped into his grandmother, whom he loved dearly. His grandmother was thrown off balance and fell to the floor breaking her hip. An ambulance came and took her to the hospital where she had surgery followed by a slow recovery. Billy was devastated. He lost fifteen pounds, developed difficulty sleeping, and became more and more anxious, withdrawn, angry, perseverative and resistive over two and a half years, moving less and less, until he would sit motionless for hours at a time. He stopped speaking. It seemed that Billy must be depressed, most likely with psychotic features and catatonia. Yet he did not respond to aggressive treatment for depression.

The neurological workup was unrevealing. His examination was remarkable for mutism, waxy flexibility and prolonged posturing. He would hold his feet off the floor just enough that a piece of paper could be slid under them and maintain this posture for hours. He had lost a good deal of weight, but with hand-over-hand feeding he managed to avoid hospitalization. There were no focal findings, no further observed seizure-like behaviors, no abnormalities on repeat EEG, cranial computed tomographic scanning, or magnetic resonance imaging, and nothing remarkable on cerebrospinal fluid (CSF) examination. Intravenous (IV) lorazepam during an EEG produced no apparent change. An interview facilitated by intravenous sodium amytal during an admission in 1992 produced no deterioration and resulted in mild improvement for three days characterized by very slow movements of his extremities to command and some ability to communicate verbally. I had followed Billy for three years and this was the first time I'd heard his voice. At the time, deterioration during an amytal interview was held to predict a neurological etiology for catatonia. Improvement portended a good prognosis with treatment

There was, however, one other remarkable development. A pizza place in a nearby town held a special dance party once a week for people over twenty-one with developmental disabilities. Participants from group homes, supported housing and families would crowd in. A DJ would play music, the patrons would dance and there would be pizza all around. Since the rest of his residential group was going to the party, Billy was brought along, too. He sat at a table with his housemates. The music started and an amazing thing happened. Billy got up and started to dance, in slow motion, but with a smile on his face. After a short time, he'd stop moving and was assisted to his seat. His residential program took him back to this club frequently in the following year and the pattern would repeat. Throughout the week Billy remained in a catatonic state with little facial expression. But when the music would start on dance party nights, he'd slowly begin to smile and dance. He'd even occasionally eat something.

Although perhaps today we would have measured autoantibodies in serum and CSF, those tests were not readily available, and the syndrome of autoimmune limbic encephalitis was not yet understood. I was convinced, though, that underneath the catatonia, Billy was still there.

After a number of new medication trials, we obtained the permission of the court to try ECT yet again, this time with increased parameters, frequency and duration. After a month of treatments three times per week, Billy spoke. He wanted to know if we had any chocolate cake. He was taken down to the cafeteria to pick out a dessert and seemed to enjoy the experience. Treatment was continued on an outpatient basis. Then one day I received a call from a staff member at his residential facility. They came downstairs one evening to find that Billy had descended the steps on his own and was in the kitchen making himself a fluffer-nutter sandwich. The staff was in tears. Billy was coming back to life. He wanted them to play music for him every evening. Sometimes he'd get up and dance for a few minutes. He gradually resumed speaking and seemed more aware of his surroundings.

At his next follow-up visit in the neuropsychiatry clinic, still being treated with weekly maintenance ECT, he shook my hand vigorously and said, "Dr. Benjamin, What happened to Reagan?"

Reagan had been the president when Billy had descended into catatonia. Mysteriously, George H W Bush was now the president. Billy
had lost eleven years of his life and was ready to pick up where
he'd left off.

Sheldon Benjamin, MD
Vice Chair for Education in Psychiatry
Director of Neuropsychiatry
Professor of Psychiatry and Neurology
UMass Chan Medical School

*The following Vignette by a former patient merits an introduction
to provide the context for his vignette*

SINGING THROUGH STUTTERING

Gene Beresin, MD, MA

A couple of years ago, I was referred a patient, Rohan, who
has an incredibly rare genetic disorder described as an autosomal
recessive neurodegenerative disorder with stuttering dysarthria,
gait impairment, dystonia and rigidity. In short, this young man,
when I first met him, he is 24, is wheelchair bound, has severe
muscle spasms of both arms and legs, with, at times, extreme pain,
inability to walk, and extreme problems talking fluidly without an
incomprehensible stutter. He routinely uses his cell phone to type
his thoughts and feelings and communicate with others.

His neurologist and primary care physicians tried virtually every
muscle relaxant known to modern medicine, though Botox and
Occupational Therapy have been mildly effective. And to compli-
cate matters, his prognosis is uncertain. Needless to say, he came in
depressed and was referred to me for therapy and treatment.

I found Rohan to be a brilliant young man and an extremely
talented poet. He was completing his college degree when I first
met with him. In addition to our agreeing to weekly psychotherapy,
I tried a number of antidepressants, and all failed to make a difference. He found that medical marijuana helped his spasms and
mood, but most of all he found great pleasure in music, attending
at least 4 musical events weekly. "Music works," he said, "better
than anything."

I am not a music therapist, but I am a musician, and we had a lot in common in terms of our musical preferences. Fortunately, he was a huge fan of music from the 60s and 70s. I asked what his two favorite songs were, and without hesitation he said, *Stairway to Heaven* and *Buffalo Soldier*. I asked if he liked to sing, and he typed, "no, not really." In that session I printed copies of both songs and proceeded to sing *Stairway to Heaven*: "There's a plant on my shelf, and some books on my wall, and I want you to sing what you see." And he responded, although reluctantly. He was totally fluid. Not a single hesitation, no stuttering at all. From then on, we sang together for many of our sessions. What was amazing to me was that if he chose not to sing and started typing, I would say, "sing it," and he stopped, gazed into my eyes, and spoke a fluid sentence. I knew that singing used other parts of the brain rather than the area used for fluent speech, but I never thought that just asking to sing would tap into those other regions. And he would be fluent without singing!

Most of our sessions have been spent enjoying clips he took of the bands he saw that week and looking at their set lists. We have a friend of mine in common. Milt Reder, MD, who is a professional musician, and plays for a Grateful Dead cover band. And he often captures a Milt solo for us to enjoy together. When we wanted to hear an original version, we would go to YouTube and see various bands playing the tune.

I asked what helped his depression the most: experiencing live music, listening to recorded music, or singing. And he said, "in that order." Why was the live music so much better? "Because it connects me with others immersed in the music."

In other sessions, he would show me his poetry. Many of these were intended to be set to music, or have music played behind them. Last year his poem, *Haiku Blues* was the winner of the Cambridge, Massachusetts Sidewalk Poetry Contest and his poem was embedded in concrete. And he complied a set of his poems into a book, each with a work of graphic art created by one of his friends.

My work with Rohan has become one of the most important times of my week. Our love of music and poetry trump any medication I can give. Our therapy is mutual. We spend our time singing, listening, and joining our spirits in our connection with live music.

We know that the music will not correct the genetic root cause of his neurological condition, though it might help. Who knows? And as he would say, who cares! What counts is surrounding ourselves in music together.

Our mutual love and connection in this musical space fosters our communal resilience.

This is all that matters.

Here is a poem I asked him to write to capture how music improves his well-being.

Music Saved My Life

I live for music

I feel it in my veins

It takes me places

Lyrics take the reigns

The notes are washing over me

To have them touch my heart

I close my eyes and see

Music in the art

All different colors, shapes and sizes

As the watercolors are dripping and splattering

I hear the music play on

I think music maybe the key to saving the world

It's a universal language

Language of love

It makes no sense when you hear it

But you get goosebumps when you do

Journeying inwards

Grooving to the sound of art and music

Through the labyrinth of life

We find ourselves

Reliving the cycle of life and death

To the center and back again

Unpeeling, unveiling the multifaceted self

That is of all

Rohan Nijhawan

Poet

Music, Memories, and Mourning

Music is an inextricable part of life. It's also intimately related to grief and mourning. My son Julian died from suicide at 32 years of age, almost one year ago. Words cannot describe the anguish and sorrow that have become central features of my life. It's been a slow and painful journey across turbulent seas of sadness and longing, a seemingly endless passage in uncharted waters. Gradually, I've come to appreciate how much music is a part of this voyage.

At first, my grief for my lost son was intolerable to the point where I couldn't bear to listen to music, let alone try to play my guitar. Just as I had lost my taste for food and my desire for sex, the simple joys of music abandoned me. For a time, I was too heartbroken to open myself to the feelings that music engenders. Hearing any song that reminded me of Julian was enough to break me down into a puddle of sobs.

Eventually, I summoned up the courage to pick up my guitar. I started playing songs we sang when Julian was young: Cat Stevens' *Moonshadow*, James Taylor's *You've Got a Friend*, Steve Goodman's *City of New Orleans*, Paul Simon's *The Boxer,* The Beatles *Hey Jude*... As I sang these songs, eyes closed, I could picture my beautiful boy smiling and singing along. I kept playing through the tears; and as I did so, I realized my broken heart was experiencing pain and joy simultaneously. It was uplifting to feel the music inside me again. It gave me strength.

At around this time, my daughter, Isabelle, put together a Spotify set list of Julian's favorite songs. They span his life and his musical tastes (which were eclectic) and they're linked to vivid memories I have of Julian listening and dancing to them. Songs like Eminem's *The Real Slim Shady*, Lil Wayne and Drake's *Right Above It*, Gloria Gaynor's *I Will Survive*, Daft Punk/Pharell Williams/Nile Rogers'

Get Lucky, Manfred Mann's *Do Wah Diddy*, Michael Jackson's *Thriller*, Swedish House Mafia's *Don't You Worry Child*, and Kevin Lyttle's *Turn Me On*.

Last summer, while walking through Fairmount Park on the way to a concert at the Mann Music Center, *Turn Me On* was playing loudly on a picnicker's sound system. I stopped in my tracks, closed my eyes, and felt Julian's spirit pulsating through me. I was filled with his presence. It was a visitation, without a doubt.

Later that summer, at a James Taylor concert on the Camden waterfront, when JT began to play *Fire and Rain*, I broke down into heavy sobs and cried my eyes out for the rest of the concert. Julian always loved JT. We went to hear him several times at that same venue – so many wonderful memories of those concerts. It was sorrowfully beautiful to be there on that warm summer night, absorbing the music and holding Julian close to me.

As time has passed, I've returned to playing and listening to music daily. I'm keenly aware of the way certain songs evoke tears while others make me smile. There's no way to predict what gets summoned from within. Recently, while driving to work, I put on one of Julian's CD mixes of his favorite songs. O-Zone's *Dragostea Din Tei* came on. I immediately started singing along, laughing loudly as I pictured Julian imitating that lip-synching Romanian kid whose YouTube video went viral in 2006: "Ma-ya-hi, may-ya-hoo, ma-ya-hah, ma-ya-ha-ha."

Then, a favorite artist releases an album that sears my soul – Bonnie Raitt's album *Just Like That* has an amazing song - *Livin' for the Ones:*

"I'm livin' for the ones who didn't make it

Cut down through no fault of their own

Just keep 'em in mind, all the chances denied

If you ever start to bitch and moan."

Sing it Bonnie. You're strumming my pain with your fingers. Thank you, thank you, *thank you!*

Tony Rostain, M.D. Chair of Psychiatry,
Professor of Psychiatry and Pediatrics, Cooper Medical
School of Rowan University; Band member, Pink Freud and the
Transitional Objects.

Music as a New Lens

A decade ago, I had the idea to invite music graduate students from our local university to perform in our mission-driven public hospital. I imagined string trios playing Mozart in the lobby and music students engaging our medical students and residents in some (ill-defined) way that would make them less depressed and more humane. I scheduled an appointment with the head of the music department to explore the idea. He was receptive. It was easy to see the advantage of playing in a central place for patients and families to enjoy; a few moments of beauty and distraction to offset the day's challenges. Then he asked me why I wanted our medical learners to interact with their music students. I explained that we recruit the most idealistic and deep feeling human beings into medicine, people who want to help and to heal, and then we proceed to train those values and sensibilities out of them. I had an instinct that exposing our trainees to music and musicians (people who devoted their lives to creating and perfecting and sharing beauty) would help them hold on to their motivation to be healers. The music director began laughing. I was taken aback. Then he asked me a question: "Do you think it's any different for musicians?" He went on:

> our students come in wanting to play music, to create meaning and beauty, and over time the system, the competition, trains that out of them. Before you know it, all they care about is playing at Carnegie Hall and signing with a record label!

He told me that he liked my idea because he thought that somehow our medical trainees might humanize their music students.

> Your students and residents are out in the community, in the real world. They interact with complex human beings with stories and backgrounds that are inaccessible to our music students. I was thinking your trainees would help motivate our students to make music that is more accessible, that makes the world a better place!

In the end, that director left his position before we could launch the music and medicine exchange. But the conversation has stayed with me. Music and medicine are each lenses to make sense of this world, to alleviate suffering, to create beauty and meaning; but lenses, if used rigidly or exclusively, force people to see certain things and stop seeing others. On the journey of professional formation, wonder and curiosity and kindness are sometimes left at the gate. We must find a way to bring them along with us, and to model them for our students. We must hold each other up with whatever gifts we have to give.

Elizabeth Gaufberg MD MPH
Associate Professor of Medicine and Psychiatry,
Harvard Medical School
Director, Cambridge Health Alliance Center for Professional and
Academic Development

Corridor Music

While working as a mental health nurse in a large hospital in the UK I struggled with low mood. The environment of the institution was depressing. The corridors were dark and littered with cigarette ends. I wondered how I had ended up working in such a place and whether I should move on to somewhere more uplifting. One day, as I walked through the building, I heard music. It was jazz. I liked what I heard and wondered where the music came from. I set out to find its source. When I followed the path of sound, I came to the end of one of the smaller corridors running off the main drag and saw a patient sitting outside the door to ward, playing a clarinet. I did not know at the time that the patient was a well-respected musician. I was captivated by the wonderful sounds he made. As I listened, I wondered who was recovering whom? The patient had become my physician. When I returned to my own ward I felt brighter, more optimistic, energized. I had just received a different kind of music therapy.

Professor Paul Crawford
University of Nottingham

Music, Addiction and Recovery

Music brings people together and is a language we share. Recovery from opioid use also has its own language. We are *all* affected by substance use disorder: personally, through family and friends, and as a society. The numbers of overdoses and deaths per year only tell part of the story. It's the people who have lived this struggle and fight for recovery every day that bring this social challenge to the surface, into our living rooms, boardrooms, schools, and in September 2018, to the stage.

The newly formed *Above the Noise Foundation* has a core mission to stomp stigma and elevate support for those in, and in need of, recovery. Two women, Kristen Williams-Haseotes and Maureen Cavanagh set out to create the first of its kind sober music festival in Pawtucket, Rhode Island at McCoy Stadium: *Recovery Fest 2018*. The event was headlined by GRAMMY-award winner *Macklemore*, with *Fitz and the Tantrums*, and other iconic New Englanders like *Livingston Taylor*. The goal? To bring together those in recovery, allies of the addicted, healthcare providers, and the musicians who care to share their talent.

It's no surprise that this epidemic is not helped by societal stigma, yet we have come very far at the same time. In 1914, the *Harrison Narcotic Tax Act* actually made it illegal for doctors to prescribe opiates for addiction, and for decades this problem has not been considered a disease, rather it has been viewed as a social misconduct issue, or moral failure.

Chronic disease is the common denominator for heroin, synthetic opioids, and prescription pill addiction. Let's look at the chronic disease diabetes: Do we stigmatize and not provide care for people in need during a diabetic crisis? Is there an "insulin equivalent" for the *brain* for opioid addiction to regulate this illness? Yes. It has become clearer that recovery is possible with maintenance treatment with the drug Suboxone. Suboxone evens out the cravings, avoids the extreme highs by weakly binding to the same receptors that bind to powerful drugs. At Recovery Fest, many posed the obvious questions: Can the music we love target that same reward center in the brain, and fulfill our dopaminergic-driven cravings? Can music tap into pleasure and memory regions and receptors in a unique and side-effect-free way?

The hope for recovery is real, thanks not only to treatment, but to the comradery and love from allies and families brought together at Recovery Fest. This gathering of thousands showed us how to turn something scary and daunting into something positive, and

how to plant the seeds of sobriety. That common language of music
made it possible for that seed to grow.

It is not a mystery that the lifestyle of the rock musician can be
non-stop, adrenaline-packed and peppered with drug use. However, as artists become role models, they can use this platform – the
stage, to promote recovery and decrease stigma. At Recovery Fest,
the musicians spoke and sang with pride in their voices, embracing
sobriety as *cool*, and as a guiding force in their lives. The synergy
of music and the message of recovery was undeniably powerful.
There was energy without substances, elation without drugs, and
all around us, so many reasons to care.

Ron Hirschberg, MD
Assistant Professor, Physical Medicine and Rehabilitation
Harvard Medical School
Director, Health and Wellness
Home Base Program for Veteran and Family Care
Director, Consultation Physiatry
Massachusetts General Hospital

An Orchestra in the Hospital

I'm an academic geriatric psychiatrist at the University of Nebraska
Medical Center (UNMC) and have worn a number of hats in my years
as a faculty member – clerkship director, resident supervisor, department chair, and of course clinician. Throughout all of these experiences I have had a strong interest in teaching my patients, students, and
colleagues stress management techniques like meditation, mindful-
ness, physical exercise, gratitude journaling, and similar things. Now, I
have the privilege of serving as the assistant vice chancellor for campus
wellness at the University of Nebraska Medical Center. When I took
on this new responsibility, I got a request of a colleague of mine to
start a "medical orchestra" at my institution. Despite being completely
inexperienced in this, I helped initiate one at UNMC. It's a joint effort
of the academic health center and our wonderful School of Music at
the University of Nebraska Omaha. Auditions were held in the summer of 2018, and the first concert of the Nebraska Medical Orchestra
(NMO) was December 5, 2018. It's no exaggeration that I was truly
astonished by the quality of that first concert! The whole audience was

just rapt. We held that concert in the lobby of our hospital, and it was fun to watch hospital visitors walk by and wonder what was going on.

Over this last year I've heard amazing anecdotes from the students, staff, and faculty who play in the NMO about the stress-relieving effects it's had, and their campus concerts definitely serve to bring joy to the standing-room only audiences. It's very heart-warming to sit in the audience and see colleagues whom you work with clinically during the day playing their cello, flute, or bass at that evening concert. Patients here too have been pleasantly surprised to attend a concert and see their doctor up on stage playing for them! I have really seen firsthand the healing power of music – both for the audience members, but equally for the performers. Some of the musicians in the NMO have formed close bonds with fellow clinicians whom they didn't know before joining the orchestra, and they get together to play duets or chamber music on their own.

Another heartwarming "side effect" of the orchestra project is a real grass-roots effort on the part of a small band of students, who formed an acapella singing group they call "Doc'Apella." It's been taking off by leaps and bounds, and the students have now sung at over a dozen venues in the last year. It's been a great benefit for the students and anyone within earshot.

As a result of this partnership between the music school and the health center campus, we are now working on a program to send musicians to do a participatory music class to a senior living facility in the area. As a geriatric psychiatrist who sees patients in local nursing homes, I'm very enthusiastic about the potential to bring some very tangible benefit to older adults, many of whom are lonely and will really benefit from the interaction and just the fun of making music. I've also been approached by several people on campus who'd like to sing in a choir, so that's the next "music and medicine" project for us. Who knows what other great projects are just around the corner? I sense we are just warming up…

Steven P. Wengel, MD
Assistant Vice Chancellor for Campus
Wellness for UNO and UNMC
Geriatric Psychiatry Division Director
University of Nebraska Omaha
University of Nebraska Medical Center

Because You Are You

For families who have engaged in, experienced, witnessed, and survived interpersonal violence and trauma, music therapy can serve as a uniquely valuable resource for coping, healing, and recovery. Music as part of a therapeutic relationship can activate and give voice to living metaphors and archetypes of emotion, transcending verbal discourse – while doing so from within a *safe-enough* working space, wherein feelings associated with traumatic material can be explored and processed from a tolerable, symbolic distance. Through music, families can discover new ways of relating to one another in more empathic, respectful, and mutually accountable ways. It can honor a person's agency and decisions, unconditionally and non-judgmentally, and allow for shared, vicarious, *here-and-now* experiences for negotiating relational dynamics in real time.

During the 2000s, as a music therapist and faculty member at a university music therapy training program, I served in a consulting role as part of a team of psychosocial professionals at a local family services organization that provided a psychoeducational counseling program for families who have experienced domestic violence and trauma. Specifically, the program was designed to provide resources for children who have witnessed or who have otherwise been exposed to any forms of violence (physical, psychological, etc.) between parents or other principal caretakers.

The program was designed in compliance with a state law that court-mandates families who have experienced domestic violence to attend a full, 12-week course of an approved, remedial psychoeducational counseling programs. My role was to collaborate with other members of the team on an inter-professional basis, integrating music therapy as an experiential, creative, artistic component of the larger, multidisciplinary structure of the program. The goal was to adhere to the curricular sequence of the program, while honoring each family members' need to explore and convey otherwise un-accessed and unexpressed thoughts and emotions and to mobilize creativity and imagination as vital, insight-oriented coping resources. In essence, it was a form of developmentally-tailored, defined-length, group music psychotherapy

Participating families attended the program on a weekly basis. Multiple families would attend simultaneously, to work in groups, together. Upon arriving, family members would be grouped developmentally according to age, comprising a young children's group, an intermediate-age children's group, an adolescent group, and a parent group. Student music therapists (under supervision), clinical supervisors, other psychosocial professionals (e.g., social workers), and myself facilitated the various groups. The structure of each group session consisted of three primary phases. First, there was a *greeting and opening experience*, which typically took the form of something musical (e.g., an improvisational "warm up," a "hello song," etc.). Second, there was a *core experience*. This involved anything from music listening, song/lyric exploration, original song composition, musical games, improvisation (often involving specifically experiences such as live, musical representation of family dynamics, or improvising music to describe action in scenes from films or television as they played with the original soundtrack silenced), and music combined with other expressive arts modalities such as drawing or movement. Third, there was a closing experience – again, which typically involved something musical).

I had the opportunity to work with each of the groups and found myself moved by what each of the groups accomplished, together. For example, in the intermediate group, I helped facilitate an experience of *soundtracking* scenes from a film involving interpersonal conflict and resolution. I genuinely appreciated how the participants took the initiative and risk within the safety of the space to create symbolically projective, esthetic forms embodying often traumatic aspects of their experience that may well have otherwise been too intimidating, too overwhelming, or simply inaccessible, via conventional verbal conversation.

I spent several consecutive weekly meetings with the members of the parent group, who chose as their shared goal to identify a way to convey unexpressed feelings and messages to their children via group songwriting. My role in the songwriting process was to employ my artistic and clinical sensibilities to suggest various options from a musical palette (e.g., choices of lyrics, melodic contour, tempo, key, harmonic/chordal accompaniment, etc.), and various ways of constructing the composition, integrating music and lyrics into a coherent song structure that honored the intentions and choices of group participants. The process challenged participants to cultivate the virtues of sensitivity, empathy, reciprocity, honesty, authenticity, trust, creativity, and imagination – while the song we were composing served as an embodiment of the group's shared originality and uniqueness and engendered a collective sense of ownership and stakeholdership for the validating gift they would share with their children.

Based upon weeks of dynamic negotiation on the elements of the song, we agreed upon a folk/rock style "anthem" written in an alternating verse-chorus structure, rooted in a major key and a triple (3/4) meter. Once completed, the parents shared the song – entitled, *Because You Are You* – publicly, "serenading" their children at a culminating gathering including all members of the program, in one room. The following comprise the lyrics of the song:

BECAUSE YOU ARE YOU

Verse One:

It takes a whole family to change what we do, and make all the wrong into right

No matter what happens, I want you to know–it isn't your fault when I fight

Chorus:

I'll always be there, I'll always be proud–You're perfect, whatever you do

I'm working to change, but no matter what, I love you because you are you

Verse Two:

I wish I could teach you what you need to know, and not have to threaten or yell

I'm trying to listen more clearly each day, so I can learn from you as well

[Chorus]Verse Three:

You are important, you matter to me, I'm grateful to know you are here

I wish you a life that's happy and full, and a home without violence or fear

[Chorus x2]

The experience of serving as a consulting music therapist in this program helped me understand how music, when engaged within a clinical context with the support and guidance of a trained music therapy professional, can be beneficial for families who have witnessed and/or survived violence and trauma in numerous ways. For the parent group, the song they wrote served as an enduring, esthetic form embodying feelings, beliefs, and values of the group, which could then be shared with their community children. It was an honor to witness the work of these families as they identified and mobilized resources available to them through the numerous relationships engendered by music.

Brian Abrams, PhD, MT-BC, LCAT
Associate Professor of Music and Coordinator
of Music Therapy
John J. Call School of Music
Montclair State University

Bye Bye Blackbird

I met L. while employed as a music therapist at an assisted living community in a suburb south of Boston. The section of the community where I worked was dedicated to residents with dementia, mostly above eighty years old, and mostly with mid-stage Alzheimer's Disease. Often, I was paired with residents that had musical abilities and/or a musical career, since I have advanced education, training, and experience as a pianist and composer. L. was one of these remarkable residents.

I was introduced to him quickly upon his entry into the community and told that he was a saxophone player. This was an obvious introduction, as he took his saxophone with him, in its case, strapped to a little metal dolly, to every meal, to every outing, to every activity. From this first meeting, it was clear that this instrument was incredibly important to him, not only giving him meaning, but also some sort of grounding.

My relationship with L. was based completely around music. Once or twice a week, I would gather a dozen residents into the great room, pull up a chair for him to sit in, and wait as he slowly put his instrument together. (When we first started this routine, he did this on his own, and as time went by and the disease progressed, I would assist him as needed.) Once his saxophone was assembled and its strap was around his neck, he would play a few scales to warm up and to signal me that he was ready to start playing. Very few words were ever spoken, nor were needed, during this routine.

For the next half hour, L. and I performed jazz standards for the residents of this community. One of us would name a piece that was in his repertoire (his family had given me a list of songs that he knew), and off we would go. What I found truly remarkable about his playing is that not only would he remember the melody of each tune – he also created short improvisations on those melodies, a skill which requires a great deal of musical knowledge as moment-to-moment awareness and creativity. These times of music-making were a high point of both of our weeks; his ear-to-ear grin after each song was the only evidence I needed.

As time went on, his playing became a bit less fluent, he forgot the names of some of the tunes, sometimes he even forgot how to play until he sat down, and I put the saxophone into his hands. But until very close to the end of his life, we made music together, entertaining the residents of this community with *Bye Bye Blackbird* (his favorite) and others. When he passed away, his family gave me the saxophone reed that he used during all of those times we played together. It sits, a treasure, on my bedroom dresser.

Trevor Berens, MT-BC, LMHC
Board Certified Music Therapist

Aphasia Blues

"We wrote this song, Aphasia Blues. Don't have all the words, oh what to do!"

Aphasia is a language disorder that can occur as a result of a stroke or head injury to an individual. The disorder impairs one's expression and understanding of language and is also commonly accompanied by emotional and psychosocial changes as well. Additionally, individuals with aphasia are prone to social isolation and exclusion. Social isolation results in a higher risk of negative health effects, compared to individuals who engage in meaningful, productive activities with others. Research has shown that human beings are naturally social creatures. Take a moment to imagine what it would be like to lose your ability to speak, to comprehend, and fully interact with the world. According to a 2016 national survey on aphasia awareness, currently around two million people in the United States are living this way.

"People we meet, they talk too quick. Gotta slow down! That does the trick!"

Few are familiar with the term, aphasia, despite the estimated number affected by the disorder. According to the same national survey mentioned above, 8.8% of people have heard of aphasia and can identify it as a language disorder. Without proper awareness and identification of this disorder, the journey toward reintegrating individuals living with aphasia back into communities can be a challenging task. Individuals with aphasia are more likely to experience isolation, often as a result of a lack of empathy and understanding of what the individual is experiencing. We've found the best way to raise awareness and provide a supportive space for those living with aphasia is through singing.

"Now there's a place I like to go. Aphasia group, they know to talk slow!"

Community aphasia choirs aim to provide meaningful interactions and experiences amongst those with this shared diagnosis. Aside from the psychosocial element, music is also a wonderful tool for recovery in aphasia therapy. Research has shown that even when individuals lose their ability to speak, their ability to sing is often retained because the right hemisphere of the brain is non-damaged. Therapeutic singing, a technique often used within aphasia choirs, is "success-oriented." Those who are engaged in singing are motivated by the emotional, and certainly in the case of the choir, social context music can provide. Therapeutic Singing can be used with all members, despite their severity, to increase participation and thus during rehearsals individuals' social and rehabilitation goals are reached.

"We rely on each other, that's what good friends do!"

The Boston University Aphasia Chorus seeks to empower its members and prioritize relationships for those living with aphasia to understand, manage, and continue to live a full-filled life despite their diagnosis. The chorus, originally founded in 2015, consists of around 25 members, many of whom have been part of the choir from the beginning. The mission of access and advocacy starts from the moment the first rehearsal begins and transforms into a reality when the chorus is in the community sharing their story. Not only has the choir performed several times within the community, but they have even written and performed an original song together. The "Aphasia Blues" continues to be a powerful way for members to share their voice through song as lyrics bring attention to the everyday challenges of communicating, while emphasizing the communal support found within the Boston University aphasia chorus. Everything changes when members are in front of a crowd. Instead of clinicians having to tell them to smile while singing, the members can't stop smiling, and with that, they bring an amazing presence to the room. Some chorus members are even brought to tears during the performance while reflecting on all the work put into each rehearsal. Singing is meant to be shared with others, and our chorus members use music and singing as an effective way to bring awareness to the disorder itself, as well as showcase the talents and abilities of the members themselves.

Delaney Mohesky
Neurologic Music Therapist Fellow
MedRhythms, Inc.

4

WAYS TO ENGAGE WITH MUSIC

We have seen throughout this book that music, either passive listening or active participation in music by playing, singing, or dancing can improve well-being. In clinical populations, musical interventions decrease anxiety, improve mood, assist emotional regulation, relieve pain, and for those with neurodegenerative disorders, improve cognition, attention, orientation, memory as well as motor functioning. But just as important, for those of us who do not have impairment, playing an instrument has preventative benefits such as reducing the risk of developing dementia in older adults (Verghese et al., 2003). In addition, for all of us, listening to music decreases anxiety, lowers blood pressure, lowers heart rate, and reduces cortisol (Panteleeva et al., 2017). Moreover, as we reflect on mutual recovery as described in Chapter 1, listening to music supports our healthcare staff by increasing empathy, preventing burnout, decreases stress and fosters resilience (Horwitz, 2018).

Now, let's take music out of a clinical framework. There are countless ways music helps us. We can use it for soothing, calming, or conversely – getting us fired up. It can inspire us, bring back memories, or help us relax and fall asleep. It can be shared by our sending tunes, playlists, or music videos to friends and loved ones. The options are limitless and each of us have our own preferences for engagement: listening to background music (I have background music on virtually all the time, unless I am watching a movie or involved with media that has its own music); playing an instrument; going to concerts; dancing – alone, or with others; writing our own songs; or joining a choir or vocal group. We can use music to amplify our study of history and cultures by listening to the music that is indigenous.

But what about children? Does playing an instrument have an impact on future development? There was a theory, substantiated by initial research that playing an instrument increases IQ – the so-called "Mozart effect." Subsequent studies disproved this. However, there have been other studies that demonstrate that when children engage in music lessons there is advancement in a range of intel-lectual skills, but studies show that these are short-lived (Chabris, 1999). The benefits of playing a musical instrument do, in fact, bestow the child with enhanced, though temporary cognitive per-formance. Long-term benefits include improved spatial skills, verbal tasks, sound processing, rhythmic awareness, and motor skills. And there is inherent enjoyment in sounding better and better and own-ing a sense of accomplishment. It can heighten pride and self-esteem. Yet many kids quit.

WHY WOULD THIS BE?

It turns out that multiple factors influence which children play an instrument and stick with it over time. It's very common for kids to start an instrument, often at the suggestion of a parent, and in short order give it up. Or they continue, reluctantly, without the pas-sion, fortitude, and dedication to persist. Often these elements of disinterest plus investable setbacks (that are expectable) lead them to throw in the towel. Others switch to a different instrument and fall in love with it, albeit a transient passion, and they eventually give up that one as well. On the other hand, some kids continue their musical studies for many years, with increasing pleasure and enthusiasm. As you can see, and most know from personal experi-ence, the variations in our relationships with music education and playing an instrument are all over the map.

The traits that distinguish the kids who persist are those who are academically inclined, have educational opportunities for music education (at home, in music schools or in their second-ary school), the support of their families, motivation and interest that fuels discipline, responsibility, and concentration and perhaps most important, good interpersonal relationships with music teachers. Often these kids come from higher socioeconomic families, though not necessarily. When considering those who continue with an instrument and those who drop out, we need to weigh in a child's personality. Those with persistence, higher executive functioning, ability to maintain a commitment, to tolerate failure and have higher frustration tolerance are likely to stick with an instrument. Anyone who has tried to learn an instrument appreciates that there is more than ample irritation, willingness to sound terrible, and for most of us, intermittent frustration, and at times anger and irritability at the length of time it takes to make progress. This is especially hard for kids, who tend to become impatient and want instant results. Yet, the more a child becomes increasingly proficient, makes fewer mistakes, learning proceeds at a higher pace and satisfaction increases. And the result enhances self-esteem, pride, and the social pleasure of playing alone or with others. It makes sense.

It's even harder for adults. How many times have you heard a friend say that they wished they never quit the piano? When they witness the personal satisfaction of others making music, they often feel that they have missed something. Indeed, they have. And some try to learn to play in mid or later life. Most adults find it more difficult and frustrating to learn an instrument than when they were younger. The same is true for learning new languages. And, in the every-day world of work, chores, maintaining a household and for some, raising children, there is little time to learn an instrument. It is perhaps easiest when one is retired, as the daily life activities required diminish greatly. But learning an instrument is a worthy cause in any case. It increases self-expression, fosters social connections, and promotes overall health and well-being. Those adults who include listening or playing music as part of daily activities have greater satisfaction with life and enhanced security. They tend to be happier, more satisfied, calm, and hopeful compared to those who do not play music regularly.

The benefits are clear. But how can we engage in music on a regular basis? Let's look at what we can do on our own and with others actively and passively.

A. ACTIVE THINGS TO DO

Active things you and your children can do with music take time, dedication, and need to incorporate your music with the rest of your life. In many cases, this is not easy until you get into the groove, and it becomes a kind of a regular part of your schedule.

Here are some tips for active participation.

1. **Encourage Your Kids To Play:** This takes a series of conversations. The younger they start the better. If you or your partner is taking up an instrument, active learning to play an instrument may become a kind of family project. Kids should be able to choose the instrument they want to pursue. I preferentially like the piano, because it has all the keys and chords visually apparent; it helps them learn to read both clefs of music (treble and bass); and, as a percussive instrument, it helps them learn rhythmic structures. If there are opportunities in school, that may be a great way to start or reinforce music education as they get to play with their friends, this reinforces the motivation. Below I will outline some practicing guidelines for kids and adults, but practice, even a short time every day is important. Making a connection with your instrument – making it feel as if it is an extension of you, even for 15 minutes daily is super important.

2. **Your playing:** I would encourage you to play as well, and I do think the piano is a good place to start, as noted above, even if you yearn to play the cello, bass, or a horn. A year or so of learning basic music principles is easiest on the piano, and if you switch, say, to the saxophone, that only plays one note at a time, by starting with the piano, you will already appreciate how the melodies outline the chord progressions, and you will have a better sense of rhythm. So just sit at the piano daily and build it into your schedule.

3. **Practicing:** Now let's look at what counts as proper practicing, and what you or your kid can do to make it interesting. Consider the style of music you ultimately want to play. I recommend beginning with classical pieces because they allow for using both hands in concert; the simple pieces are relatively

easy to learn; and they allow for learning to read as well as play. If your ultimate interest is rock, blues, pop, country, jazz, or any other form, you can and probably should pick a piece you really like in addition to a classical piece. There are some tunes at a beginner's level for every genre.

Some key principles, of practicing (Duke et al., 2009):

a. First, remember, it is not about the amount of time you choose, say 30 minutes a day. 30 minutes of bad practicing is not helpful. What helps is playing whatever you are working on correctly, slowly, and getting the notes and the timing correct.

b. Use a metronome to keep in time.

c. Start slow and then speed up to the recommended tempo of the exercise or piece.

d. I like to break practicing down into: scales and exercises, played slowly, correctly and in time. Hannon is the gold standard. There are also some excellent practice etudes in the style.

e. Then choose two pieces you really like: a simple classical piece; and a piece in the style you really want to play – say a blues.

f. I would spend some after you do your exercises, etudes, and pieces, to just sit and play. Play anything! Play along with a tune you really like from an online music app, like Spotify.

g. Work with a teacher you really like. You can find them at your secondary school (public or private), local music schools, or those who offer private lessons. There are even teachers you can get online, though I don't think it is as effective as having your teacher sitting with you. But your relationship with your teacher cannot be over-emphasized. They not only show you how to do things correctly, but remembering that music is a social enterprise, the attachment with your teacher and their encouragement, support, guidance, and practical demonstration is critical.

h. If you want to learn on your own, though less personal, YouTube has a huge number of sites that provide instruction in virtually every instrument. Some have a whole series of lessons starting with beginners; while other, for those of you who know an instrument – at least the basics – and can pick up learning new tunes, scales, riffs, and techniques that you cannot pick up on your own. Such instructional material used to be sold as DVDs (and I probably have about 75 or more), but now you can either download them, keep them in an onsite library, or subscribe with a YouTube account and create several instructional playlists on your own. I do this for guitar, as it is far easier for me to play new material with a guitar and watching a screen than using the piano.

i.   Online play along material is also available in a number of apps. For example, you can buy an inexpensive app that has drums, bass, piano, or guitar, and play along, or leave one instrument out so you can fill in with your chosen instrument. There are also apps that you can import a piece of music, say a complex Charlie Parker or Oscar Peterson solo (with an impossibly large number of notes), and slow it down as slow as you like, without changing the pitch. In the old days, when you slowed down an LP or a tape, the pitch dropped, and you were in a different key. With modern technology, you can learn the most complex solos in virtually any style of music by simply slowing it down, then learning sections of it until you master it. Imitation and learning a solo note for note, either from a digital app or from a written transcription is not "cheating." The best way to learn the subtle inflections, chords, back up parts, or improvisational lines, is by memorizing the leads of great musicians. This will give you ideas you can then use in other pieces of music.

j.   Suzuki, famously said "you don't have to practice every day, only the days that you eat." In other words, unless you are sick, you need to sit down at the piano – even a few minutes.

4. **Play With Others:** As we have emphasized in this book, you cannot underestimate the power of playing music with others (Bostic et al., 2019). And this means setting up regular get-togethers in which everyone can play, sing, drum, or dance.

Some groups that I have known use apps that allow everyone to have lyrics and chords; others provide sing-along books, self-made or bought; while others go around the room with each participant choosing the tune, or the drum circle rhythm. Allow the tunes, lyrics, instruments to be available for anyone to select. This was the essence of the hootenannies of the 1960s and are as welcome today. In some concerts, the lead singer welcomes audience participation, and a vast crowd of people, are singing with the band. Sometimes the lyrics are on a big screen, other times, many folks who know that band and all their popular tunes need no lyrics, and others unfamiliar with them, clap, or dance along with everyone else. Both venues are the foundation of the community music noted in Chapter 1, and are typically uplifting, engaging, and socially connecting. Even sad music makes folks happy (Sloboda & Justin, 2001)! That is well known listening to the blues. It has been shown that sad music, evokes multiple emotions that intensify pleasure – through releasing endorphins and prolactin, both associated with gratification and relaxation (Huron, 2011). Sad music also implies that one is not alone, because others in the room are enjoying it as well.

For others, most spiritual groups have choirs you can join that participate in regular services. Other places of worship have choirs that sing on a regular basis. There are often community organizations that have choral groups from highly professional ones to informal groups. Many of these, including a cappella groups can be found online in your community. If you can't find one, start one! You do not have to be an experienced singer or choir leader to do this, and if you are intimidated in leading this mission, putting in a tweet on your local community site may well turn up someone who has a lot of experience. The main point is taking initiative to be part of a social musical group.

B. PASSIVE THINGS TO DO

We have seen that passive listening to music has numerous benefits, perhaps not as many as active singing, playing, or dancing, but listening, as we have seen, promotes well-being in many ways, by regulating emotions, relieving pain, improving cognition, such as autobiographical memory and attention.

Here are some ideas about how you can benefit from passive listening.

1. **Attend Live Musical Events:** While it is easiest to go to concerts, many venues do not provide a sense of community. You could go with friends who are fans of the performers. But better, I think, is attending outdoor concerts, festivals, and block parties. At festivals and block parties, not only can you hear a wide range of music, but you are also part of a community, and the social integration enhances your pleasure in the music.

2. **Share Playlists:** During the COVID lockdown, adolescents achieved mood regulation and social cohesion by sharing playlists (Chiu, 2020). Listening to music together, when combined with talking proved extremely effective in combatting loneliness. My family shared a "Quarantine Spotify Playlist," during the beginning of the COVID lockdown with each family member contributing a song. It was not only important in keeping us connected, but I learned about artists I never knew before, and I am sure the same was true for others. So, creating and sharing playlists is a great way of not only connecting with others, but introducing music friends and family may not have heard.

3. **Watch and Share Musical YouTube Videos:** More than ever, YouTube serves as a powerful search engine. In fact, it is likely second only to Google. You can find almost any musical artist or song using YouTube. For music, it compares with, and some feel it is better than the most commonly used musical apps, e.g., Spotify, Apple Music, Amazon Music. Many young people use YouTube as it does not require subscriptions for premium services as many music apps do. If you and family or friends use an online platform, such as Zoom or many others and share screens, a YouTube video of a music video can be shared. It also can be shared on social media. The bottom line is this: you can enjoy, connect, and learn about new music through sharing with online media. While it may not take the place of live concerts or festivals, it provides an immediate alternative.

8. **Listen to Music Together:** We noted earlier in this book that young people share similar music with their parents. This seems counterintuitive for adolescents seeking to separate, differentiate, and become autonomous as they struggle to find their own identity. Yet most share musical tastes with their families. Listening together, for holidays, celebrations, after dinner, or sadly during times of loss, is a valuable means of relaxation, regulating emotions and bonding with family members.

9. **Learning About New Musical Artists and Genres:** Many of us have not had much exposure to certain artists, venues, or styles of music. For example, jazz standards may not be in the musical repertoire of many young people. Playing music for them, exposing them to music they have never heard may be an enlightening experience. I have learned about many new artists from my kids, as it is so hard to keep up with current music, particularly when I am focused on jazz and blues. The great thing about new artists is that music apps and YouTube often have many of their songs or instrumentals, and we can all learn from each other.

10. **Background Music:** We have seen that background music can significantly reduce anxiety and pain in a wide range of settings including pre- and post-operative care, in labor and delivery, and during surgical procedures. It is even more effective if the music is preferred by the patient awaiting an operative procedure. The literature on background music at work, and for kids doing their homework is mixed. For many it has a positive effect on productivity, concentration and overpowering unwanted noise. Yet for others, it is an unwanted distraction. There are children with Attention Deficit Hyperactivity Disorder (ADHD) who do better work, paradoxically, when they listen to hip-hop or rap, and though this seems paradoxical, perhaps it is the regularity of the beat, bass and drums that somehow helps them focus. Background music may be a way to help us relax, to improve our work skills, or conversely be an unwanted interruption. My best suggestion is to experiment and see what works for you.

Engaging in music, either actively or passively may be a powerful way to enhance well-being in your life. I would encourage you to get involved both actively and passively, but by all means engage with music! I am confident you will find the right fit for your health and lifestyle.

5

HOW PROFESSIONALS CAN USE MUSIC TO IMPROVE WELL-BEING

Professionals can use music in several settings – in hospitals, nursing homes and assisted living facilities, at home, particularly for palliative or hospice care. Let's first look at the research that documents the efficacy of music interventions, both passive and active in a number of environments. Then we should think about the challenges that professionals face in providing what should be a cost-effective, non-pharmacologic approach for alleviation of psychological stress, pain, and anxiety.

PERI-OPERATIVE SETTINGS

Spintge nicely summarizes the many studies using music in pre-operative settings, in the operative rooms themselves, and in post-operative units and found that music reduces anxiety, pain, and stress. He notes that there is strong evidence for the efficacy of musical interventions in surgery of all sorts, dentistry, and neonatal care. Further, he points out that many studies have demonstrated physiological signs of benefits, including reduced heart rates, lowered blood pressure, improved sleep, and reduced post-operative confusion. He calls this kind of musical intervention Anxioalgolytic Music (AAM) (Spintge, 2012). Substantiating his review, a meta-analysis of 92 RCTs, including 7,385 patients having a wide range of surgical procedures, demonstrated that musical interventions compared with controls, before, during and after surgery found that musical interventions significantly decreased anxiety compared with controls (those who did not have musical interventions), and substantial reductions in pain for those who had musical interventions during their general anesthesia (Kühlmann et al., 2018).

While there is a wealth of studies regarding the effectiveness of music in operative situations, let's look at three common surgical interventions: neurosurgery, cardiac surgery, and cataract procedures.

In a review of seven studies, it was noted that music was effective in reducing anxiety, pain, heart rate and blood pressure following neurosurgical procedures (Kwong et al., 2022). An analysis of 20 studies looking at patients undergoing cardiac surgery, in the post-operative period music sessions was associated with reduced anxiety and pain. Multiple days of music intervention reduced anxiety up to 8 days post-operatively (Kakar et al., 2021). Patients who were undergoing cataract surgery had pre-operative music with earphones for 20 minutes and a control group did not. The group listening to pre-operative music had significantly lower levels of anxiety and lower rates of pain compared with the group that did not listen to music both during the procedure and upon completion of the cataract surgery (Guerrier et al., 2021).

These and many other studies have consistently demonstrated that music interventions peri-operatively have a profound impact on anxiety and pain. It is very common for surgeons to play background music during procedures, but it's hard to determine how much of this is for them, for the anesthesia staff, for nurses, or for the patients themselves. Frankly, it doesn't matter. We have seen earlier in this book that the principle of mutual recovery assists both the patients as well as the caregivers.

I had two knee replacements by the same surgeon, and had spinal anesthesia, so I was awake for much of the time. I clearly recall he and the staff singing along to the music. From my perspective, I appreciated how calm it made all of us feel to be enjoying the same music throughout the surgery. In fact, as he was closing up, having removed my knee and provided a mechanical replacement, he turned to me and said, "you know, Gene, I'd like to play you my favorite song. Are you up for it?" I nodded. Then he put on Fred Astaire, singing "They Can't Take That Away From Me" from the original recording. And (and I swear this really happened and I was not delirious), the nurses and orthopedic fellows began dancing around the operating table. It was like a scene from a TV show. What was most valuable, besides the irony of tune chosen, was the feeling in the operating room. Everyone was enjoying themselves, and I can't convey how this enhanced my sense of well-being. As a thank you a few weeks later, I sent my surgeon an album of Fred Astaire singing his greatest hits, including this tune, with Oscar Peterson playing piano. He loved it. And I listened to it over and over as I endured the pain of physical therapy, for my new knee. For anyone having a knee replacement, the pain of rehab is awful, and the music, the memory of the OR and the dancing, all helped me get through the pain of rehabilitation.

INTENSIVE CARE UNITS

The intensive care unit (ICU) is a terrifying place both for patients and their families. It houses patients with severe, life-threatening conditions, and is experienced with uncertainty both by the clinicians as well as the patients. In short, it is not a comfortable place for anyone. In a very comprehensive review of several studies, intervention sessions of 20–30 minutes by a music therapist, in the ICU was significantly helpful in decreasing anxiety, pain, agitation, lowering anesthesia, and sedative medications, as well as decreasing feelings of discomfort, improving sleep quality and diminishing the propensiity propensity for delirium (Chen et al., 2021).

Substantiating this review, in one study comparing adult patients in an ICU receiving 20-minute music therapy consisting of a combination of musical songs and instrumental music chosen by the therapist, with patients who did not receive this intervention, those who did responded with reduced anxiety and improved physiological parameters, including temperature, pulse, respiratory rate, blood pressure, and oxygen saturation (Chahal et al., 2021).

PEDIATRIC SETTINGS

Children and adolescents are particularly to sensitive and responsive to music therapy. In an extensive review of the effectiveness of music therapy, music medicine and other music-based interventions, there was considerable positive value of music in a wide range of populations including children with autism spectrum disorder, physical disabilities, pediatric cancer, epilepsy, mental illness, and kids undergoing medical procedures, and neuroreabilitation regardless of the setting -- all noting decreases in anxiety, pain and stress (Stegemann et al., 2019).

Palliative care at home was studied for children, "hospital-at-home" with music therapists providing sessions at home. The families felt less isolated yet connected to each other through the work of the music therapist (Steinhardt et al., 2021). Palliative care for pediatric patients has had positive impact in terms of improving well-being and the quality of life.

Despite the positive value of music interventions for children and adolescents, in a survey of music therapists working in pediatric medical settings in the United States, the authors found an alarming shortage of workforce and funding. The results indicated 1 certified music therapist for every 100 beds. One-third of the respondents to the survey (118 Board-certified music therapists working in pediatric settings) were the only music therapist in their setting, and half of the surveyed positions were funded by philanthropy. They also found that the call for music interventions was determined by priorities based on acuity, with palliative care and pain the most common top demands. More than half of the music therapists worked in ICU settings, hematology/oncology, or neonatal ICUs (Knott et al., 2020). This study is alarming and demonstrates the need for more music therapists available to help kids, and moreover that funding sources should be garnered from the healthcare system beyond philanthropy.

NURSING HOMES

The residents of nursing homes are generally elderly individuals who cannot be taken care of at home, either because of cognitive or physical disabilities. Most older people do not relish the idea of leaving the comfort of their homes, daily contact with family, and being in a familiar environment in which they feel safe and comfortable. Despite frequent resistance, many families must make the difficult decision to place their loved ones in nursing homes. Once established in a nursing facility, unless severely cognitively compromised, residents often make friends, and hopefully have group activities. Yet the range of staffing, programs for shared community engagement, and individual attention is extremely varied if present at all.

Musical interventions have been helpful for nursing home residents, particularly in group activities. Overall well-being for diverse residents may be particularly effectively by group music-making. Several studies have focused on group singing and its improving well-being. In one study, singing, rhythm-based activities with percussion instruments, and listening to live performances produced well-being (Paolantonio et al., 2020).

Music therapy in nursing homes relieves depression and improving well-being in those with dementia (Ray & Götell, 2018).

TREATMENT OF CANCER

I cannot think of any illness dreaded more than cancer. What could be worse than the fear of dying compounded with the dread of chemotherapy and radiation? While many cancers are treatable, virtually all individuals who live with a diagnosis of cancer experience the pain of uncertainty, anxiety, stress, and depression. These emotional consequences of cancer only add to the physical problems associated with surgery, chemotherapy, and radiation.

Music intervention is helpful for both adults and children undergoing treatment for cancer. In adults, music therapy can improve anxiety, depression, stress, and pain, along with overall psychological well-being, physical symptom distress and the quality of life (Köhler et al., 2020).

In pediatric cancer, receptive music and active music therapy is associated with a significant reduction in psychological distress and overall improvement in feelings of well-being (Facchini & Ruini, 2021). In acute hospital settings, music therapy administered for children treated for cancer can improve mood and morale (Wong et al., 2021).

It is clear that music interventions are helpful in multiple settings, and for adults, children, and families. The question raised in this chapter, is what can professionals do to improve well-being? The answer is clear – provide more music therapy, music medicine and group music activities. Yet, who are the professionals that would provide this? Most clinicians in the healthcare system in the United States are not trained in musical interventions. Music therapists are often funded by state departments of mental health, Medicare, and insurance companies. Yet as we have seen, in the United States there is only approximately 1 music therapist per 100 beds – surely a shortage in workforce, given the evidence-base for efficacy, and when music therapy is used, likely a cost-savings in terms of medications and therapeutic interventions for a variety of conditions, including anxiety, pain, sleep, muscular dysfunction and cognitive decline. And their funding is largely through philanthropy.

What can professionals do? I have been working in a large general hospital for close to 43 years. I have never heard of a request to recruit music therapists. In my hospital, they are largely used in pediatrics, and are totally supported by philanthropy. I am confident that this is true in many other hospital systems of care. What we can do is advocate for inclusion of music therapists as a core part of our medical and surgical teams. If they cannot be funded by insurance, federal or state funding, perhaps certified music therapists can provide workshops to train medical and allied health professionals to learn and use music medicine. I would prefer to have active music therapy, music medicine and group music intervention programs, but it may be the best we can do to start is to include music medicine as part of our training of medical, pediatric, and surgical clinical staff.

6

CHALLENGES FOR ENGAGEMENT
IN MUSIC

CHALLENGES IN CLINICAL SETTINGS

We have presented evidence that music therapy, music medicine, and community music have powerful beneficial effects on your physical and emotional states in medical and surgical units in hospitals, dental suites, nursing homes, and in your own home for palliative or hospice care. But many clinical settings do not have a music therapist as a core member of the team. What can you do if you want to include music intervention in your clinical care? After all, the standard of care in virtually all settings is collaborative. You have a say, indeed, a vested interest, in how your condition will be treated. Here are the challenges for incorporating music interventions as part of your care plan:

1. There may not be a music therapist, music medicine program or community program in your healthcare facility. You should ask your primary attending physician for a music component in your treatment plan. The challenge is whether their facility has a music therapist affiliated.

2. If there is music medicine as part of your peri-operative care (waiting room, operating theater, recovery room), you should consider bringing in your preferred music for your personal listening device. Bring your music on a thumb drive, or as a

playlist on your smart phone. The challenge will be to find the person on the team who will include this in your care plan, should it not be a routine procedure.

3. If your family member is in a nursing home on in your home care, how can you enlist a music therapist to become active and provide services? The challenge is whether you go an association of music therapists and have this discussion or try and contact someone privately. This, of course, likely depends on whether you have the means to pay privately for services or find out if services are covered by your insurance plan or by a national or local agency.

4. If you have a chronic condition such as cancer, or an orthopedic problem that needs ongoing rehabilitation you could see what availability a private music therapist has to accommodate your needs. Long-term illnesses merit long-term relationships.

5. You might want to establish a music intervention program in a healthcare facility that does not have one. This would require your approaching the patient care office and contacting a local or national music therapy group as many have advocates. This is a way you can help change your system of care.

CHALLENGES IN ENGAGING IN MUSIC ALONE OR WITH OTHERS

Listening to or playing music is not without its physical, logistic, or emotional dangers. I would like to present some examples of the challenges many of us face when engaging with music. Let me begin by noting that not everyone has the same challenges. Just as well-being is not the same for all of us, engaging with music is highly individualized. Let's look at the challenges in two major realms, listening and playing.

A. CHALLENGES WHEN LISTENING TO MUSIC

There is increasing evidence that listening to loud live music regularly and over time can cause hearing loss. This is a significant risk for teenagers (Petrescu, 2008). In addition, listening on personal music devices, e.g., headphone, ear buds, can also result in significant hearing loss (Engdahl & Aarhus, 2021). The mechanism for the hearing loss, or tinnitus (ringing or buzzing in the ears) is damage to the hair cells in the cochlea and other components of this important structure of the inner ear (Royster, 1995). This was particularly true using loud personal music devices.

Celebrities are the most vital sources of promoting consumer products. Some studies have shown that music celebrities endorse food products that are high in sugar and nutrient poor. This may have a negative impact on children and teenagers who admire such artists (Bragg et al., 2016). The same case may be seen when celebrities promote bluetooth headphones or ear buds for listening to music.

We are all hostages to digital media. Consider how many devices you have in your homes – smart phones, Ipads, tablets, computers, and TVs. Many of these devices, including, headphones or ear buds, are often used by children and adolescents while doing their school-work. Background music, particularly preferred music, improves attention and academic performance, despite the concerns of many parents (Kiss & Linnell, 2021). However, this may not be true for all students, and we need to consider how it may actually be a distraction for some.

Listening to music when driving may be dangerous. If you look at the literature on this, we find mixed reviews. In general, the consensus is that music is distraction for all of us, especially new teenage drivers. However the situation is more complex that simply concluding that music is altogether distracting. It turns out that when you consider standard deviations in speed, lane crossing frequency, mental work load (the focus and concentration on driving), and the heart rates of drivers, rock music produces a negative impact on these variables, whereas lighter music maybe actually improve driving performance and arousal (awareness of the driving situation). Studies also show that driver personality has a major influence – in other words drivers who have the personality of rule breaking tend to be more distracted than those who are more obedient and conformist, rather than those who tend to take risks. Thus, the influence of the genre of music in combination with the temperament of the driver is the right way to approach the challenge of what music (if any) to listen to when driving (Wen et al., 2019).

Music can have a negative impact, particularly on youth, if is overstimulating, triggers painful memories of a failed relationship, floods a vulnerable person with negative emotions, particularly associated with past traumas.

B. CHALLENGES WHEN PLAYING MUSIC

Most of us play at different levels of intensity and frequency. Some, with the highest playing time are professional musicians, or close to it. For these experienced players, there are numerous challenges. Many experience pain, such as discomfort in the back, shoulder, arm wrist, or hand, depending on the instrument. Many musicians experience chronic pain (Fishbein et al., 1988).

Playing Alone

I might add that this may not just be true for professional musicians. There are considerable physical challenges for any of us playing a new instrument. I play the guitar and have done so since I was about 13. But I only played finger picking style (Delta and Piedmont Style as exemplified by Mississippi John Hurt, Reverend Gary David, Blind Blake, and others. I also played in the style of Merle Travis, Chet Atkins, and Mark Knopfler). Acoustic guitars are generally light and easy to hold, even the large ones. During the COVID pandemic, I decided to take up blues guitar and bought a Les Paul that weighs a lot. In short order I had wrist, joint and arm pain, no matter how I tried to play the blues (Schuppert & Wagner, 1966). Shortly thereafter, I bought what is called a semi-hollow body jazz guitar, that is super light, and easy to play. The take-home message of this is that we all need to be aware that there are occupational hazards of playing certain instruments, and we need to learn how to hold them, how to sit, what kind of chair or bench to use, and other ergonomic considerations. Playing a new instrument may merit physical considerations, lest you risk tendonitis, joint pain, back pain, or other physical symptoms.

Playing an instrument for experienced musicians is not without emotional challenges. Even professional musicians report performance anxiety, fears, depression, and sleep problems. This is common, and some seek treatment for their emotional pressures.

Most of us are not professional musicians. There are significant challenges for those of us who are just starting out with a musical instrument, and those who have some experience but are either learning a new instrument, or more likely trying out a new genre of music.

We considered beginning students and the challenges of practicing in Chapter 4. For anyone taking up a new instrument, particularly adults, many experience frustration, short attention span, lack of patience, the need for discipline (yet wanting instant results), and probably the most difficult emotion to tolerate – shame when heard by others and in your view, as my current teacher says, "sound stinky."

Learning brand new skills is not easy. It is hard to see how things will turn out. The major challenge is to be tolerant of your incompetence (especially if you are competent in other areas of life), and learn to be persistent. Most of us, resist even approaching the instrument, because the experience of learning can, at times, be so emotionally taxing. The skills of playing are compounded by the necessary ability to read music, at least in a rudimentary way, learning rhythmic structures, and keeping in time.

And for those of us who are already proficient in some genres of music, learning new styles and techniques may be just as challenging. I pretty good at playing blues, rock, country, and ragtime. My band covers many tunes I can play with a fair amount of fluidity. But now I am taking piano lessons to learn jazz and improvisation. Trying to play a totally different genre when I already can play other material is particularly frustrating. In fact, it is awful! For those who don't know, traditional pop, rock and country music is based on the root (the note based on the key you are playing in) and the 5th. So, in the key of C, that would be C and G. In jazz, the core notes are the third and the seventh note of the scale, and those define the chords. So, in the key of C, that would be E and B or B flat. Your basic chords leave out the root and 5th. This means that everything thing I learned and played all my life is totally changed into seeing and hearing things in a new way. And as I fumble around, sounding "stinky," it is beyond exasperating and intolerable to feel as though I never played before. Further, in most rock, pop, blues and country, there is minimal improvisation. We call the breaks, solos, and they are pretty simple, straight forward, even though they leave room open for exquisite lines. Jazz improvisation is a totally different animal. When I play (or try to play), it is as though I have hit a wall. I just don't know what to play, even after playing piano since I was a little kid.

Playing With Others

Playing with others is among the most rewarding experiences in music. It fosters expertise in listening, enhancing the material of other musicians (making them sound even better), communicating with others through your contribution, and above all, feeling the power of music to make interpersonal connections, and producing a piece in which the whole is greater than the sum of its parts. It is an act of group creation and enhances the well-being of all.

But playing with others comes with its own challenges – different for all, but nonetheless at times problematic. Naturally, some players will be more experienced and versatile than you. This can make you feel inferior, and at worst, incompetent. Once you feel the lack of confidence, it typically makes your feel self-conscious, inhibited, and play worse. A player who feels secure, whether experienced or a beginner, plays better.

There are other challenges: knowing where you are in the tune; keeping time; maintaining an awareness of how loud, up front, or conversely, how understated you need to be to allow for a balance of all the players; tolerating your mistakes – and better how to make a mistake into a leading tone that is followed by one that fits the harmony.

All these challenges require three skills: humility, the ability to listen and self-expression. Effective group music requires the challenge to elaborate and play off of the contribution of another (even if you don't care for it), and, by listening, respond in kind so that your part adds something new that adds something to the piece.

7

OVERCOMING CHALLENGES AND FUTURE DIRECTIONS

OVERCOMING CLINICAL CHALLENGES

We have seen the many challenges involved in establishing music therapists as core members of medical, dental, surgical, and residential teams. The numbers speak for themselves. There is a huge shortage of certified music therapists to meet the clinical needs of the conditions that benefit from music therapy, music medicine and community music.

I think our challenge is two-fold.

First, we need to educate our healthcare clinicians about the clinical benefits afforded by music interventions. As I have shown, music interventions substantially help improve cognitive and motor functioning, as well as decreasing pain, anxiety, stress, and loneliness. They also have physiological benefits for our patients. Furthermore, we need to help our clinicians appreciate that through mutual recovery and caring for the caregivers, they too will benefit by decreasing burnout and improving their well-being.

Music therapy components should be a core part of the burgeoning programs in well-being for healthcare professionals, including meditation, yoga, sleep hygiene, nutrition, and exercise. This is a win-win situation.

But how do we do this? As professionals, we can begin by advocating for music intervention in grand rounds and workshops in all of our specialties and establishing affiliations between our local and national music therapy organizations and the national organizations of physicians, nurses, and allied health professionals. We begin with knowledge, awareness, and connection. At this point in time, music interventions are not close to being on the radar of our service chiefs, no less front-line workers.

We also need to educate our hospital officers and healthcare insurance companies about the cost-savings of music therapy. This will require more studies of efficacy, as well as cost-benefit and quality improvement analyses to demonstrate that coverage will save insurers and hospital systems of care substantial costs.

Second, we need to ally with our patients and members of the community and lobby for increasing the workforce of music therapists to meet future service needs. I hope that we could expand music education and music therapy programs from the secondary school level to college curricula. Music therapists will need education both as performers as well as healers. I have no doubt that this career track will be very appealing to many students. This larger workforce would be beneficial to patients and to caregivers as noted above.

OVERCOMING PERSONAL CHALLENGES

In the last chapter, I noted the many challenges of playing an instrument for the first time, of expanding one's repertoire by learning new styles and techniques on an instrument and playing with others. These personal challenges can be addressed in the following ways:

1. Practice your first instrument daily, even for a short time, and keep your expectations low in terms of how quickly you will become proficient.

2. If you are expanding your repertoire, and are learning new skills and technique, keep your expectations low and keep in mind how long it took you to learn the basics of what you already know. Also, keep up with your old, established skills, as this will reinforce your self-esteem, improve your confidence, reduce frustration, and remind you that you have already mastered material. Play a piece or two of your familiar tunes when practicing.

3. When playing with a group, whether a beginner or experienced player, keep the focus off yourself, and use the community experience to be a part of everyone's sense of resilient connection and well-being. Remember it is the group experience that counts, not what you or any single member is doing when playing together.

4. Listen, listen, listen! Make a playlist of the tunes you want to learn, and use it as background music, when you are working, when you drive, or when you are just laying low and relaxing. It is critical to have the music you want to play in your head as much as possible. The more you listen to music, the more you hear – the harmonic movement, the construction of improved lines, the subtle rhythmic structures, and more.

5. Maintain a close, warm relationship with your teacher. They are there not only to give you a musical education, but to provide support, encouragement, and reinforce your joy in learning.

Finally, although this book was designated as Music as part of the Arts in Health, music need not simply be used for clinical or one's personal educational experiences. Music has been cherished by all cultures and people of all ages as long as we humans (and perhaps other species) have inhabited this planet. It is our true salvation – healing ourselves and mending others, enriching relationships, enlightening our sense of self and identity in a world with others, transcending loneliness and isolation, and at times setting ourselves in rhythmic motion. Beyond simply using music for a particular purpose in society, sometimes we just want to listen or play music for its own sake. It is a transcendental experience be a part of creating or listening to something beautiful.

Let me end with this challenge: Enjoy the artists and tunes you already know, and please experiment with taking in new music. Feel it, absorb it. It need not serve any other function than to make you happy.

REFERENCES

American Music Therapy Association. (n.d.). Retrieved April 26, 2022, from https://www.musictherapy.org/about/musictherapy/

Bare, L. C., & Dundes, L. (2004). Strategies for combatting dental anxiety. *Journal of Dental Education, 68*(11), 1172–1177.

Bernatzky, G., Strickner, S., Presch, M., Wendtner, F., & Kullich. (2012). What is music, health and wellbeing and why is it important? In R. MacDonald, G. Kreutz, & L. Mitchell (Eds.), *Music, health & wellbeing* (pp. 3–7). Oxford University Press.

Blood, A. J., & Zatorre, R. J. (2001). Intensely pleasurable responses to music correlates with activity in brain regions implicated in reward and emotion. *Proceedings of the National Academy of Sciences, 98,* 11818–11213.

Boer, D., & Abubakar, A. (2014). Music listening in families and peer groups: Benefits for young people's social cohesion and emotional well-being across four cultures. *Frontiers in Psychology, 5,* 392. https://doi.org/10.3389/fpsyg.2014.00392. PMID: 24847296; PMCID: PMC4021113.

Bonde, L. O. (2011). Health musicking: Music therapy or music and health? A model, eight empirical examples and some personal reflections. *Music and Arts in Action,* (Special issue: Health Promotion and Wellness) *3,* 120–140.

Bostic, J. Q., Schlozman, S., Pataki, C., Ristuccia, C., Beresin, E. V., & Martin, A. (2003). From Alice Cooper to Marilyn Manson: The significance of adolescent antiheroes. *Academic Psychiatry, 27*(1), 54–62.

Bostic, J. Q., Thomas, C. R., Beresin, E. V., Rostain, A. L., & Kaye, D. L. (2019). Make a joyful noise: Integrating music into child psychiatry evaluation and treatment. *Child and Adolescent Psychiatric Clinics of North America, 28*(2), 195–207. https://doi.org/10.1016/j.chc.2018.11.003

Bradt, J., Dileo, C., & Potvin, N. (2013). Music for stress and anxiety reduction in coronary heart disease patients. *Cochrane Database of Systematic Reviews, 12*, 1–104.

Bragg, M. A., Miller, A. N., Elizee, J., Dighe, S., & Elbel, B. D. (2016). Popular music celebrity endorsements in food and nonalcoholic beverage marketing. *Pediatrics, 138*(1), e20153977. https://doi.org/10.1542/peds.2015-3977

Callahan, K., Schlozman, S., Beresin, E., & Crawford, P. (2017). The use of music in mutual recovery: A qualitative pilot study. *Journal of Applied Arts & Health, 8*(1), 103–114.

Cao, S., Sun, J. J., Wang, Y., Shao, Y., Sheng, Y., & Aiguo, X. (2016). Music therapy improves pregnancy-induced hypertension treatment efficacy. *International Journal of Clinical and Experimental Medicine, 9*(5), 8833–8838.

Carr, C., d'Ardenne, P., Sloboda, A., Scott, C., Wang, D., & Priebe, S. (2012). Group music therapy for patients with persistent post-traumatic stress disorder: An exploratory randomized controlled trial with mixed methods evaluation. *Psychology and Psychotherapy,* (2), 179–202. https://doi.org/10.1111/j.2044-8341.2011.02026.x. Epub 2011 Jun 20. PMID: 22903909.

Chabris, C. F. (1999). Prelude or requiem for the 'Mozart effect.' *Nature, 400*, 826–827.

Chahal, J. K., Sharma, P., Sulena, & Rawat, H. C. L. (2021). Effect of music therapy on ICU induced anxiety and physiological parameters among ICU patients: An experimental study in a tertiary care hospital of India. *Clinical Epidemiology and Global Health, 11*(1–6). https://doi.org/10.1016/j.cegh.2021.100716

Chanda, M. L., & Levitin, D. J. (2013). The neurochemistry of music. *Trends in Cognitive Sciences, 17*(4), 180–193.

Chang, Y. S., Chu, H., Yang, C. Y., Tsai, J. C., Chung, M. H., Liao, Y. M., Chi, M. J., Liu, M. F., & Chou, K. R. (2015). The efficacy of music therapy for people with dementia: A meta-analysis of randomised controlled trials. *Journal of Clinical Nursing*, *24*(23–24), 3425–3440. https://doi. org/10.1111/jocn.12976. Epub 2015 Aug 24. PMID: 26299594.

Chen, Y. F., Chang, M. Y., Chow, L. H., & Ma, W. F. (2021). Effectiveness of music-based intervention in improving uncomfortable symptoms in ICU patients: An umbrella review. *International Journal of Environmental Research and Public Health*, *18*(21), 11500. https://doi.org/10.3390/ ijerph182111500

Chiu, R. (2020). Functions of music making under lockdown: A trans-historical perspective across two pandemics. *Frontiers in Psychology*, *11*, 616499. https://doi.org/10.3389/fpsyg.2020.616499

Chuang, C. H., Chen, P. C., Lee, C. S., Chen, C. H., Tu, Y. K., & Wu, S. C. (2019). Music intervention for pain and anxiety management of the primiparous women during labour: A systematic review and meta-analysis. *Journal of Advanced Nursing*, *75*(4), 723–733. https://doi. org/10.1111/jan.13871. Epub 2018 Nov 11. PMID: 30289556.

Clift, S., Hancox, G., Morrison, I., Hess, B., Kreutz, G., & Stuart, D. (2010). Choral singing and psychological wellbeing: Quantitative and qualitative from English choirs in a cross-national survey. *Journal of Applied Arts and Health*, *1*(1), 19–34.

Cooke, M., Chaboyer, W., Schluter, P., & Hiratos, M. (2005). The effect of music on preoperative anxiety in day surgery. *Journal of Advanced Nursing*, *52*(1), 47–55.

Crawford, P., Lewis, L., Brown, B., & Manning, N. (2013). Creative practice as mutual recovery in mental health. *Mental Health Review Journal*, *18*(2), 55–64.

Curtis, M. E., & Bharucha, J. J. (2010). The minor third communicates sadness in speech, mirroring its use in music. *Emotion*, *10*(3), 335–348.

Dick Clark quotes. (2022). BrainyQuote.com, BrainyMedia Inc. Retrieved May 30, 2022, from https://www.brainyquote.com/quotes/dick_clark_ 133272

Donaldson, S. I., & Ellardus van Zyl, L. (2022). PERMA+4: A framework for work-related well-being, performance, and positive organizational psychology. *Frontiers in Psychology*, *12*, 817244. https://doi.org/10.3389/fpsyg.2021.817244

Duke, R., Simmons, A., & Cash, C. (2009). It's not how much: It's how. *Journal of Research in Music Education*, *56*, 310–321.

Engdahl, B., & Aarhus, L. (2021, Jan–Dec). Personal music players and hearing loss: The HUNT cohort study. *Trends in Hearing*, *25*, 23312165211015881. https://doi.org/10.1177/23312165211015881. PMID: 34181492; PMCID: PMC8245669.

Erikson, E. (1993). *Childhood and society*. Norton Books.

Facchini, M., & Ruini, C. (2021). The role of music therapy in the treatment of children with cancer: A systematic review of literature. *Complementary Therapies in Clinical Practice*, *42*, 101289. https://doi.org/10.1016/j.ctep.2020.101289

Fancourt, D., & Finn, S. (2019). *What is the evidence on the role of the arts in improving health and well-being? A scoping review.* Health Evidence Network (HEN) Synthesis Report 67, World Health Organization Regional Office for Europe Copenhagen, p. 29.

Fishbein, M., Middelstadt, S., Ottati, V., Straus, S., & Ellis, A. (1988). Medical problems among ICSOM musicians: Overview of a national survey. *Medical Problems of Performing Artists*, *3*, 1–8.

García González, J., Ventura Miranda, M. I., Requena Mullor, M., Parron Carreño, T., & Alarcón Rodriguez, R. (2018). Effects of prenatal music stimulation on state/trait anxiety in full-term pregnancy and its influence on childbirth: A randomized controlled trial. *Journal of Maternal-Fetal and Neonatal Medicine*, (8), 1058–1065. https://doi.org/10.1080/147670 58.2017.1306511. Epub 2017 Apr 3. PMID: 28287005.

Geretsegger, M., Elefant, C., Mössler, K. A., & Gold, C. (2014). Music therapy for people with autism spectrum disorder. *Cochrane Database of Systematic Reviews*, (6), CD004381. https://doi.org/10.1002/14651858. CD004381.pub3

Geretsegger, M., Mössler, K. A., Bieleninik, Ł., Chen, X. J., Heldal, T. O., & Gold, C. (2017). Music therapy for people with schizophrenia and schizophrenia-like disorders. *Cochrane Database of Systematic Reviews*, *5*(5), CD004025. https://doi.org/10.1002/14651858.CD004025.pub4

Guerrier, G., Bernabei, F., Lehmann, M., Pellegrini, M., Giannaccare, G., & Rothschild, P. R. (2021). Efficacy of preoperative music intervention on pain and anxiety in patients undergoing cataract surgery. *Frontiers in Pharmacology, 12*, 748296. https://doi.org/10.3389/fphar.2021.748296

Hackney, M. E., & Earhart, G. M. (2009). Effects of dance on movement control in Parkinson's disease: A comparison of Argentine tango and American ballroom. *Journal of Rehabilitation Medicine, 41*, 475–481.

Hawkley, L. C., & Cacioppo, J. T. (2010). Loneliness matters: A theoretical and empirical review of consequences and mechanisms. *Annals of Behavioral Medicine, 40*(2), 218–227. https://doi.org/10.1007/s12160-010-9210-8

Hays, T., & Minichiello, V. (2005). The meaning of music in the lives of older people: A qualitative study. *Psychology of Music, 33*(4), 437–451.

Horwitz, E. B. (2018). Humanizing the working environment in health care through music and movement. In L. O. Bonde & T. Theorell (Eds.), *Music and public health: A Nordic perspective* (pp. 187–199). Springer International.

Huron, D. (2011). Why is sad music pleasurable? A possible role for prolactin. *Musicae Scientiae, 15*(2), 146–158.

Iasiello, M., Bartholomaeus, J., Jarden, A., & Kelly, G. (2017). Measuring PERMA+ in South Australia, the state of wellbeing: A comparison with national and international norms. *Journal of Positive Psychology and Wellbeing, 1*(2), 53–72.

Kakar, E., Billar, R. J., van Rosmalen, J., Klimek, M., Takkenberg, J. J. M., & Jeekel, J. (2021). Music intervention to relieve anxiety and pain in adults undergoing cardiac surgery: A systematic review and meta-analysis. *Open Heart, 8*(1), e001474. https://doi.org/10.1136/openhrt-2020-001474

Karapetsas, A. V., & Laskarki, R. M. (2015). Coping with loneliness through music. *Encephalos Journal, 52*, 10–13.

Kiss, L., & Linnell, K. J. (2021). The effect of preferred background music on task-focus in sustained attention. *Psychological Research, 85*, 2313–2325. https://doi.org/10.1007/s00426-020-01400-6

Knott, D., Biard, M., Nelson, K. E., Epstein, S., Robb, S. L., & Ghetti, C. L. (2020). A survey of music therapists working in pediatric medical settings in the United States. *Journal of Music Therapy*, 57(1), 34–65. https://doi.org/10.1093/jmt/thz019

Koelsch, S., & Jancke, L. (2015). Music and the heart. *European Heart Journal*, 36, 3043–3048.

Köhler, F., Martin, Z. S., Hertrampf, R. S., Gäbel, C., Kessler, J., Ditzen, B., & Warth, M. (2020). Music therapy in the psychosocial treatment of adult cancer patients: A systematic review and meta-analysis. *Frontiers in Psychology*, 11, 651. https://doi.org/10.3389/fpsyg.2020.00651. Front;11:2095. PMID: 32373019; PMCID: PMC7179738.

Kwong, K. C. N. K., Kang, C. X., & Kaliaperumal, C. (2022). The benefits of perioperative music interventions for patients undergoing neurosurgery: A mixed-methods systematic review. *British Journal of Neurosurgery*. https://doi.org/10.1080/02688697.2022.2061421

Kühlmann, A. Y. R., de Rooij, A., Kroese, L. F., van Dijk, M., Hunink, M. G. M., & Jeekel, J. (2018). Meta-analysis evaluating music interventions for anxiety and pain in surgery. *British Journal of Surgery*, 105(7), 773–783. https://doi.org/10.1002/bjs.10853. Epub 2018 Apr 17. PMID: 29665028; PMCID: PMC6175460.

Kushnir, J., Friedman, A., Ehrenfeld, M., & Kushnir, T. (2012). Coping with preoperative anxiety in cesarean section: Physiological, cognitive, and emotional effects of listening to favorite music. *Birth*, 39(2), 121–127. https://doi.org/10.1111/j.1523-536X.2012.00532.x. Epub 2012 May 17. PMID: 23281860.

Landis-Shack, N., Heinz, A. J., & Bonn-Miller, M. O. (2017). Music therapy for posttraumatic stress in adults: A theoretical review. *Psychomusicology*, 27(4), 334–342. https://doi.org/10.1037/pmu0000192

Leciere, C., Viaux, S., Avril, M., Achard, C., Chetousni, M., Missonnier, S., & Cohen, D. (2014). Why synchrony matters during mother-child interactions: A systematic review. *PLoS One*, 9(12), e113571. https://doi.org/10.1371/journal.pone.0113571

Leubner, D., & Hinterberger, T. (2017). Reviewing the effectiveness of music interventions in treating depression. *Frontiers in Psychology*, 8, 1109. https://doi.org/10.3389/fpsyg.2017.01109

Levitin, D. J. (2006). *This is your brain on music: The science of a human obsession* (p. 119). Penguin Group.

Linnemann, A., Kappert, M. B., Fischer, S., Doerr, J. M., Straher, J., & Nater, U. M. (2015). The effects of music listening on pain and stress in the daily life of patients with fibromyalgia syndrome. *Frontiers in Human Neuroscience, 9*, 434. https://doi.org/10.3389/fnhum.2015.00434

Loersch, C., & Arbuckle, N. L. (2013). Unraveling the mystery of music: Music as an evolved group process. *Journal of Personality and Social Psychology, 105*(5), 777–798. https://doi.org/10.1037/a0033691

Loveday, C., Woy, A., & Conway, M. A. (2020). The self-defining period in autobiographical memory: Evidence from a long-running radio show. *Quarterly Journal of Experimental Psychology, 73*(11), 1969–1976. https://doi.org/10.1177/1747021820940300

MacDonald, A. R. (2013). Music, health, and well-being: A review. *International Journal of Qualitative Studies on Health and Well-being, 8.* https://doi.org/10.3402/qhw.v8i0.20635

MacDonald, R., Kreutz, G., & Mitchell, L. (2012). What is music, health and wellbeing and why is it important? In R. MacDonald, G. Kreutz, & L. Mitchell (Eds.), *Music, health & wellbeing* (pp. 3–7). Oxford University Press.

Mehr, S. A., Singh, M., Knox, D., Ketter, D. M., Pickens-Jones, D., Atwood, S., Lucas, C., Jacoby, N., Egner, A. A., Hopkins, E. J., Howard, R. M., Hartshorne, J. K., Jennings, M. V., Simson, J. H., Bainbridge, C. M., Pinker, S., O'Donnell, T. J., Krasnow, M. M., & Glowacki, L. (2019). Universality and diversity in human song. *Science, 366*(6468), eaax0868. https://doi.org/10.1126/science.aax0868

Miranda, D. (2013). The role of music in adolescent development: Much more than the same old song. *International Journal of Adolescence and Youth, 18*(1), 5–22. https://doi.org/10.1080/02673843.2011.650182

Molnar-Szakacs, I., & Overy, K. (2006). Music and mirror neurons: From motion to 'e'motion. *Social Cognitive and Affective Neuroscience, 1*(3), 235–241. https://doi.org/10.1093/scan/nsl029

Mushtaq, R., Shoib, S., Shah, T., & Mushtaq, S. (2014). Relationship between loneliness, psychiatric disorders and physical health? A review on the psychological aspects of loneliness. *Journal of Clinical and Diagnostic Research*, 8(9), WE01–WE4. https://doi.org/10.7860/JCDR/2014/10077.4828

Nakata, T., & Trehub, S. E. (2004). Infants' responsiveness to maternal speech and singing. *Infant Behavior and Development*, 27, 455–464.

North, A. C., Hargreaves, D. J., & O'Neill, S. A. (2000). The importance of music to adolescents. *British Journal of Educational Psychology*, 70, 255–272.

Osman, S. E., Tischler, V., & Schneider, J. (2016). 'Singing for the brain': A qualitative study exploring the health and well-being benefits of singing for people with dementia and their carers. *Dementia*, 15(6), 1326–1339.

Panteleeva, Y., Ceschi, G., Glowinski, D., Courvoisier, D. S., & Grandjean, D. (2017). Music for Anxiety? Meta-analysis of anxiety reduction in non-clinical samples. *Psychology of Music*, 1–15.

Paolantonio, P., Cavalli, S., Biasutti, M., Pedrazzani, C., & Williamon, A. (2020). Art for ages: The effects of group music making on the wellbeing of nursing home residents. *Frontiers in Psychology*, 11, 575161. https://doi.org/10.3389/fpsyg.2020.575161

Petrescu, N. (2008). Loud music listening. *McGill Journal of Medicine*, 11(2), 169–176.

Rafieyan, R., & Ries, R. (2007). A description of the use of music therapy in consultation-liaison psychiatry. *Psychiatry (Edgmont)*, 4(1), 47–52.

Raglio, A., Zaliani, A., Baiardi, P., Bossi, D., Sguazzin, C., Capodaglio, E., Imbriani, C., Gontero, G., & Imbriani, M. (2017). Active music therapy approach for stroke patients in the post-acute rehabilitation. *Neurological Sciences*, 38(5), 893–897. https://doi.org/10.1007/s10072-017-2827-7. Epub 2017 Jan 30. PMID: 28138867.

Ray, K. D., & Götell, E. (2018). The use of music and music therapy in ameliorating depression symptoms and improving well-being in nursing home residents with dementia. *Frontiers in Medicine (Lausanne)*, 5, 287. https://doi.org/10.3389/fmed.2018.00287

Reddick, B. H., & Beresin, E. V. (2002). Rebellious rhapsody: Metal, rap, community, and individuation. *Academic Psychiatry*, 26(1), 51–59.

Royster, J. D. (1995). Noise-induced hearing loss. In J. L. Northern (Ed.), *Hearing disorders* (3rd ed., pp. 177–189). Allyn and Bacon.

Ruud, E. (1997). Music and the quality of life. *Nordic Journal of Music Therapy*, (2), 86–97. https://doi.org/10.1080/08098139709477902

Särkämö, T., Tervaniemi, M., Laitinen, S., Numminen, A., Kurki, M., Johnson, J. K., & Rantanen, P. (2014). Cognitive, emotional, and social benefits of regular musical activities in early dementia: Randomized controlled study. *Gerontologist*, *54*(4), 634–650. https://doi.org/10.1093/geront/gnt100. Epub PMID: 24009169.

Schmid, W., & Ostermann, T. (2010). Home-based music therapy: A systematic overview of settings and conditions for an innovative service in healthcare. *BMC Health Services Research*, *10*, 291. https://doi.org/10.1186/1472-6963-10-291

Schuppert, M., & Wagner, C. (1966). Wrist symptoms in instrumental musicians: Due to biomechanical restrictions? *Medical Problems of Performing Artists*, *11*, 37–42.

Seligman, M. E. P. (2002). *Authentic happiness*. Simon & Schuster.

Seligman, M. (2018). PERMA and the building blocks of well-being. *The Journal of Positive Psychology*, *13*(4), 333–335. https://doi.org/10.1080/17439760.2018.1437466

Sihvonen, A. J., Sarkamo, T., Leo, V., Tervaniemi, M., Altenmuller, E., & Soinila, S. (2017). Music-based interventions in neurological rehabilitation. *Lancet Neurology*, *16*, 648–660.

Silverman, M. J. (2003). The influence of music on the symptoms of psychosis: A meta-analysis. *Journal of Music Therapy*, *40*(1), 27–40.

Simon, H. B. (2015). Music as medicine. *American Journal of Medicine*, *128*(2), 208–210. https://doi.org/10.1016/j.amjmed.2014.10.023. Epub 2014 Oct 19. PMID: 25448175.

Sloboda, J. A., & Justin, P. N. (2001). Psychological perspectives on music and emotion. In P. N. Justin & J. A. Sloboda (Eds.), *Music and emotion: Theory and research* (pp. 71–104). Oxford University Press.

Spintge, R. (2012). Clinical use of music in operative theaters. In R. MacDonald, G. Kreutz, & L. Mitchell (Eds.), *Music, health & wellbeing* (pp. 276–286). Oxford University Press.

Stegemann, T., Geretsegger, M., Phan Quoc, E., Riedl, H., & Smetana, M. (2019). Music therapy and other music-based interventions in pediatric health care: An overview. *Medicines (Basel)*, 6(1), 25. https://doi.org/10.3390/medicines6010025

Steinhardt, T. L., Mortvedt, S., & Trondalen, G. (2021). Music therapy in the hospital-at-home: A practice for children in palliative care. *British Journal of Music Therapy*, 35(2), 53–62. https://doi.org/10.1177/13594575211029109

Stige, B. (2012). Health musicking: A perspective on music and health as action and performance. In R. MacDonald, G. Kreutz, & L. Mitchell (Eds.), *Music, health & wellbeing* (pp. 183–195). Oxford: Oxford University Press.

Thoma, M. V., La Marca, R., Brönnimann, R., Finkel, L., Ehlert, U., & Nater, U. M. (2013). The effect of music on the human stress response. *PLoS One*, 8(8), e70156. Published 2013 Aug 5. https://doi.org/10.1371/journal.pone.0070156

Tseng, P. T., Chen, Y. W., Lin, P. Y., Tu, K. Y., Wang, H. Y., Cheng, Y. S., Chang, Y. C., Chang, C. H., Chung, W., & Wu, C. K. (2016). Significant treatment effect of adjunct music therapy to standard treatment on the positive, negative, and mood symptoms of schizophrenic patients: A meta-analysis. *BMC Psychiatry*, 16, 16. https://doi.org/10.1186/s12888-016-0718-8

Verghese, J., Lipton, R. B., Katz, M. J., Hall, C. B., Derby, C. A., Kuslansky, G, Ambrose, A. F., Sliwinski, M., & Buschke, H. (2003). Leisure activities and the risk of dementia in the elderly. *New England Journal of Medicine*, 348(25), 2508–2516. https://doi.org/10.1056/NEJMoa022252. PMID: 12815136.

Volpe, U., Gianoglio, C., Autiero, L., Marino, M. L., Facchini, D., Mucci, A., & Galderisi, S. (2018). Acute effects of music therapy in subjects with psychosis during inpatient treatment. *Psychiatry*, 81(3), 218–227. https://doi.org/10.1080/00332747.2018.1502559. Epub PMID: 30351238.

Wen, H., Sze, N. N., Zeng, Q., & Hu, S. (2019). Effect of music listening on physiological condition, mental workload, and driving performance with consideration of driver temperament. *International Journal of*

Environmental Research and Public Health, 16(15), 2766. https://doi.org/10.3390/ijerph16152766

Wijk, H., Neziraj, M., Nilsson, Å., & Ung, E. J. (2021). Exploring the use of music as an intervention for older people living in nursing homes. *Nursing Older People*. https://doi.org/10.7748/nop.2021.e1361

William James Quotes. (n.d.). *BrainyQuote.com*. BrainyQuote.com Web site. Retrieved May 30, 2022, from https://www.brainyquote.com/quotes/william_james_38252

Wong, K. C., Tan, B. W., Tong, J. W. K., & Chan, M. Y. (2021). The role of music therapy for children undergoing cancer treatment in Singapore. *Healthcare*, 9, 1761. https://doi.org/10.3390/healthcare9121761

Zhang, Y., Cai, J., Zhang, Y., Ren, T., Zhao, M., & Zhao, Q. (2016). Improvement in stroke-induced motor dysfunction by music-supported therapy: A systematic review and meta-analysis. *Scientific Reports*, 6, 38521. https://doi.org/10.1038/srep38521

URL LINKS

Five notes to rule them all: the power of the pentatonic scale. https://www.percussionplay.com/five-notes-to-rule-them-all/. Accessed April 25, 2022.

Happiness is key to overall wellness: Dali Lama. (2013). https://economictimes.indiatimes.com/magazines/travel/happiness-is-key-to-overall-wellness-dalai-lama/articleshow/24629450.cms?from=mdr. Accessed April 25, 2022.

https://www.bbc.com/future/article/20180928-the-surprising-truth-about-loneliness. Accessed April 26, 2022.

https://www.multivu.com/players/English/8294451-cigna-us-loneliness-survey/. Accessed April 26, 2022.

https://www.wbur.org/news/2018/05/25/cvs-hold-music. Accessed April 27, 2002.

INDEX